# Emergency Pr[obscured] d
# Fi[obscured]



*Muriel Skeet*

SRN FRCN
International Nursing and Health
Services Consultant

Formerly:
Chief Nursing Officer
British Red Cross Society and
Joint Committee of the Order of
St John of Jerusalem and British Red Cross;
Chairman, Nursing Advisory Committee
League of Red Cross Societies;
President, Commonwealth
Nurses' Federation

Blackwell Scientific Publications
OXFORD LONDON EDINBURGH
BOSTON MELBOURNE

Editorial offices:
Osney Mead, Oxford OX2 0EL
8 John Street, London WC1N 2ES
9 Forrest Road, Edinburgh EH1 2QH
52 Beacon Street, Boston
Massachusetts 02108 USA
214 Berkeley Street, Carlton
Victoria 3053 Australia



First published 1981

Printed and bound in
Great Britain by
Henry Ling Ltd at the
Dorset Press, Dorchester

DISTRIBUTORS
USA
Blackwell Mosby Book
Distributors
11830 Westline Industrial Drive
St Louis, Missouri 63141

Canada
Blackwell Mosby Book
Distributors
120 Melford Drive, Scarborough
Ontario M1B 2X4

Australia
Blackwell Scientific Book
Distributors
214 Berkeley Street, Carlton
Victoria 3053

British Library
Cataloguing in Publication Data
Emergency procedures and first aid for nurses.
1. Emergency nursing
I. Skeet, Muriel
610.73′61 RT120.E4

ISBN 0–632–00594–7

# Contents

# Contributors

*Ursula Brown* BSc (Hons), SRN, JBCNS Cardiothoracic Course Cert, DN(Lond), RCNT
Clinical Teacher, The Brompton Hospital, London

*Veronica Chapman* SRN, RNT, DN(Lond)
Nurse Tutor, Princess Alexandra School of Nursing, The London Hospital

*Joan Darwin* SRN, RNT
Director of Nurse Education, Kingston and Richmond Area Health Authority

*Kathy Edwards* SRN, RSCN, SCM
Senior Nursing Officer, Chelsea Hospital for Women, London

*Donald Macleod* FRCS Ed
Surgeon, Bangour General Hospital, Broxburn, West Lothian, Scotland

*Elizabeth McAlister* SRN, SCM, QIDN(Cert), RCNT, DN
Nursing Officer, Surgical Area, Royal Victoria Hospital, Belfast, Northern Ireland

*Joan Markham* SRN, SCM, STD, HV, DN
Formerly Area Nursing Officer, Kingston and Richmond Area Health Authority

*Muriel Skeet* SRN, FRCN
International Nursing and Health Services Consultant, formerly Chief Nursing Officer, British Red Cross Society

*Brenda Slaney* SRN, DN(Lond), OHNCert, Tech Teachers Cert, Dip in Social Studies
Principal Advisory Tutor in Occupational Health Nursing, Royal College of Nursing of the United Kingdom

*Elaine Ward* SRN, SCM, MTD
Principal Nursing Officer, Queen Charlotte's Hospital for Women, London

# Preface

Every citizen of our contemporary world any day and in any country can find himself or herself in dire need of the knowledge and skills of first aid. None more so than the nurse.

On or off duty, at work, attending sporting events, motoring, on holiday, in a restaurant or just walking along a street she or he can meet up with a situation requiring the know-how of an emergency procedure. To have to stand by and do nothing because one does not know what to do or how to carry out the procedure which is urgently required can be a devastating and an unforgettable experience—the purpose of this book is to prevent that happening.

However, what are thought to be correct emergency procedures today may not be considered to be so tomorrow: over the past few years, for example, we have witnessed more than one change in the treatment of burns, bites, poisonings and methods of resuscitation and transporting casualties. A wide variety of opinions exists on many aspects of first aid. I am fully aware therefore that not all procedures described in this book will win the total support of all experts in the field. The contents, however, do represent not only approved teachings in some of the country's centres of excellence but also some practices and findings learnt by the authors from first-hand experience. And for that, I maintain, there is no substitute.

With the exception of the two main life-saving procedures—artificial ventilation and external cardiac massage, which are covered at the beginning of the book—each chapter has been written as a complete guide in the particular field it covers. Although this inevitably results in some overlap and repetition, it is my hope that it will increase the value of the work as a source of quick reference.

It is my great pleasure to thank all those colleagues who assisted or advised and the contributors for their willing cooperation and for sharing their expertise in this way.

I am most grateful to Churchill Livingstone for permission to reproduce the table on page 171 from *Emergencies in Medical Practice* by C. A. Birch and those on pages 250 and 251 from one of my own publications *Manual for Disaster Relief Work.*

I should also like to thank the *British Medical Journal* and Professor W. H. Rutherford for allowing me to quote from *Surgery of Violence,* and the Pergamon Press for permission to use material from *Disasters: Medical Organisation* by T. L. Baillie and J. Boer.

My thanks are due to the Voluntary Aid Societies for their help with the section on moving and transporting casualties. To these and to the many other people who have advised and guided me in emergency situations I extend my warm appreciation.

*May 1981* *Muriel Skeet*

# Introduction

First aid is the immediate and temporary care given to a person who has been injured or who has become suddenly ill. Its essential purpose is to provide such care as will benefit patients preparatory to their receiving definitive treatment.

## DIMENSIONS OF THE PROBLEM

### Trauma

In the United Kingdom, more people under the age of forty die from accidents than from any one fatal disease. Drivers, particularly adolescents and young men, are at highest risk. Eighty-five per cent of all patients who suffer spinal cord injury, for example, are young men between the ages of eighteen and twenty-five. The crucial period for this type of injury is the first 4 hours after the accident. Skilful and knowledgeable care both at the site and from the site are of extreme importance: they can make the difference to a casualty of minimum or no disability and severe life-long impairment.

Serious burns not only may affect underlying structures such as tendons, joints, muscles, nerves, blood vessels and even bones by direct thermal damage but can have through their systemic effect serious and lethal consequences.

Uncontrolled bleeding leading to hypovolaemic shock can kill. The treatment of the traumatic patient must therefore be directed towards these effects and towards the prevention of infection—which may readily occur when body defences are breached.

### Medical conditions

Since the turn of this century, giant strides have been made in controlling communicable diseases. Some, such as smallpox, have been eradicated; others, such as diphtheria and measles, greatly reduced. But new killers have appeared. Heart attacks are the single leading cause of fatalities in this country. Of those people who die from a heart attack, half never reach a hospital alive, and two-thirds are dead within 2 hours. Diabetic coma undetected and untreated remains as fatal as ever. Patients who suffer cerebrovascular accidents, poisoning and acute respiratory crises require immediate care. Slender time margins can again mean the difference between disability or full recovery and between life and death. And those time margins depend upon one variable—adequate and immediate care.

## Psychiatric problems

Mental illness has emerged as one of the leading disablers of the twentieth century. Most families have need of some understanding of mental health these days and often have to cope with emotional crises. Rising death rates among adolescents and young adults since the early 1960s have contributed to the doubling of the homicide and suicide rates in Great Britain.

Drug abuse, an increasingly frequent companion to mental illness, has meant an increase in the number of patients who suffer overdoses. Of growing national concern is the number of abused children, victims of parent and family problems in today's stressful age. These children experience physical and emotional trauma, often requiring sophisticated management techniques. Early referral is dependent upon early recognition.

## Environmental risks

There are numerous environmental factors that impinge upon health: the pace of modern living; the insecurity brought about by redundancies; high-rise blocks of flats; air pollution; deafening (literally) noise; substandard housing and the use of hazardous appliances and pieces of equipment at work and during recreation.

It is no longer feasible to shrug off the victims as solely responsible for their own conditions. Professionals and informed lay people recognise that they are the responsibility of the whole community: the general public must contribute in the development of adequate responses to the whole range of environmental problems with which we are faced.

## RESPONSES TO THE PROBLEM

Until recently in the United Kingdom the prevailing attitude was that responsibility for the victims of injury began in the casualty department of the local hospital. The cause of the injury (or illness), the circumstances surrounding or leading to the event and how the patient was transported to hospital were all secondary considerations.

Since the early 1960s this has changed. Figures at that time indicated that at least 20 per cent of all accident and coronary deaths could be avoided if prompt treatment were available at the scene and during transport to hospital. Translated into terms of an average town of 50,000–60,000 people, this meant the saving of 20 to 40 lives and the prevention of hundreds of people becoming disabled. In national cost terms it meant a saving of something like £5 million. The impact of such statistics caused a reappraisal of the availability of people trained in first aid. Prevention and safety also took on new meanings.

Four areas have, in consequence, received attention. First, modification of the environment includes: the manufacture of safer materials for clothing (especially children's nightwear); the installation of occupational safety measures; housing reforms; and the passing of laws such as those affecting the taking of alcohol and driving. The second is an approach aimed to bring knowledge and skills to the individual: swimming lessons for children; advanced driving instruction for motorists; and the like. The third is an emphasis on health education, particularly in relation to the effects of diet, exercise and smoking. The fourth entails the establishment of an adequate emergency response system in the form of trained lay first-aiders, especially throughout industry.

## THE SCOPE OF LAY FIRST-AIDERS

The lay first-aiders at work or at home are restricted to a defined role in emergency care. They must stay within established guidelines and perform only those procedures they have been trained to do. They must know their own limitations. These will be determined not only by the level of training they have received but by self-awareness of their abilities. Additional care of the casualty by a health professional must always follow the first aid which has been given by a lay person.

## NURSES AND FIRST AID

Nurses have the additional responsibility of being able to render first aid themselves. Accidents will happen. There are several thousands in Great Britain every year. Many are fatal; even more result in permanent injury, scarring, or disability. All bring suffering. Unfortunately nurses have a reputation for having only a sketchy knowledge of first aid, yet with their commitment to saving lives, their training to act promptly and their gift for improvisation, they could well be masters in this field. This book aims to set them in the right direction for becoming so.

CHAPTER 1

# The Place of First Aid in Emergency Care

First aid is the skilled application of accepted principles of treatment on the occurrence of an accident or in the case of sudden illness using those facilities or materials available at the time. It is the approved method of treatment until the casualty is removed, if necessary, to hospital or to a site where appropriate skills and equipment are available.

First aid is given to:

- sustain life
- prevent the condition from becoming worse
- promote recovery

The person rendering first aid must:

- assess the situation
- arrive at a dignosis for each casualty
- give immediate and adequate treatment, bearing in mind that a casualty may have more than one injury and that some casualties will require more urgent attention than others
- arrange without delay for transport of a casualty to hospital according to the seriousness of the condition

## INITIAL ACTION

**1.** Be calm and take charge. Give confidence by talking to, listening to and reassuring the conscious casualty.

**2.** Check:

- the safety of the casualty and of yourself
- the breathing
- for bleeding
- whether conscious

**3.** Get others to help. Tell them what to do; if necessary, send for ambulance, police, fire service, or other medical help.

## DIAGNOSIS

The history of the incident must be taken into consideration and an examination made to determine the signs and symptoms and level of consciousness of each casualty.

## TREATMENT

Sustain life.
  Clear airways and give emergency resuscitation if necessary.
Prevent the condition from becoming worse.
  Cover wounds.
  Immobilise fractures, large wounds and any injured part of the body.
  Place the casualty in a correct and comfortable position.
Promote recovery.
  Reassure.
  Give any other treatment needed.
  Relieve pain if possible.
  Handle gently and carefully at all times.
  Move as little as possible.
  Protect from extremes of temperature.

The casualty should be conveyed at once to a hospital if necessary, to suitable shelter, or to his or her own home. If to hospital or surgery, a brief written note, without abbreviations, setting out clearly what has been done and what treatment or drugs or both have been given should accompany the patient.

## GENERAL PROCEDURES FOR EMERGENCY CARE

The 5 general procedures which provide the overall framework for administering emergency care are:

**1.** Survey the situation.

**2.** Determine the nature and severity of injuries, illness or presenting problems.

3. Administer appropriate first aid.
4. Notify authorities and arrange transport.
5. Complete follow-up care.

Although for the majority of emergencies, this order may be adhered to, sometimes a change will better suit the situation. If, for example, there is someone else who can notify the appropriate authorities and arrange transport, this should be done before the completion of the necessary first aid procedures.

## Survey the situation

Pertinent information should be collected and interpreted by the first-aider. The amount of time spent on this will depend upon answers to:

How apparent are the presenting problems?
How life-threatening are the presenting problems?
How much is already known about the casualty or patient?
How life-threatening are the dangers of the environment?

### Observation

When arriving at the scene of an accident or sudden illness, the environment should be quickly scanned. This can be undertaken in a very few moments if the cause or underlying cause is apparent. This is particularly important if the patient is unconscious and alone. An emergency may involve more than one person, for example, a car accident or an outbreak of food poisoning.

Observation, based on the cause, will help the first-aider to categorise the types of emergency. Falls and crashes will most likely lead to musculoskeletal injuries, head injuries and internal bleeding. Electric shock, drowning, poisonous gases will mean respiratory emergencies. Fire will precipitate concern for burns and asphyxia. By quickly observing, the first-aider can often prepare for appropriate action.

### History of the event

Not all injuries or illnesses, however, can be easily observed. Questioning of the victim, his or her companions or bystanders is often necessary. If the patient is conscious, the history can be collected by direct questioning: What happened? If the patient is unconscious or in no state to answer questions, a history may be taken from someone who saw what happened. It is often necessary, when this method is the only recourse, to limit the story and ensure that relevant facts only are given. People will *want* to talk to relieve their own shock and anxiety.

**History of the patient**

The first-aider should ask direct questions, for instance, How do you feel? and not leading questions like Do you think you are going to faint? Baseline data, including recent medication taken, whom to contact, should be collected as soon as is practicable. If the patient is found unconscious it is wise to check for diabetic or steroid card, medic-alert bracelet and the like.

Obviously none of this must be allowed to delay getting on with first aid procedures, but a quick survey of this type will help to decide priorities and may also prevent important complications.

## Determine nature and severity of the emergency

In determining the nature and severity of an emergency, *nature* means the type, such as cardiac, pulmonary, trauma. Sometimes there is an overlap: trauma, for instance, may lead to a cardiopulmonary emergency. Each is dealt with according to classification, in subsequent chapters.

In this context, *severity* must be seen as the estimated risk to life or the graduation of a minor injury to a major one. A sprain, for instance, may be a severe one, but it will not kill. The relative seriousness of each type of injury and emergency is also dealt with in each chapter.

Decisions regarding priorities as well as appropriate treatments can then be based on this knowledge.

**Examination of the patient**

To determine both the nature and the severity of the injury or illness, examination of the patient should be carried out systematically.

*Check for vital signs*

breathing (listen and observe rise and fall of chest if necessary)
colour of skin (for dark-skinned people, note the palms of the hands, soles of feet and lips)

circulation (presence or absence of pulse at the carotid artery)
pupils (dilated and no reaction to light if circulation is ineffective)

These signs will give the first-aider information which is vital. From them it is possible to tell if there is cardiac or pulmonary arrest or both. Both threaten life and are therefore given first priority. They are dealt with in detail in Chapters 2 and 3.

*Check for severe bleeding*

Bleeding will be obvious when it occurs from external wounds on exposed surfaces of the body. It may not be obvious if it occurs under clothing or from the part of the body facing the ground. The possibility of serious internal bleeding must also be considered when signs and symptoms of severe shock are apparent after trauma. Excessive loss of blood can cause life-threatening shock in only a few minutes after injury. Severe bleeding therefore must take high priority and be dealt with immediately. Methods of how to do so are given in subsequent chapters, principally 4, 5, 6, 7 and 8.

*Check for internal poisoning*

Poisoning can cause death almost immediately. According to the amount and type of chemical taken, prompt intervention may mean the difference between life and death. General indications of poisoning include empty containers, burns or stains in and around the mouth and depressed breathing and circulation. The subject is dealt with in more detail in Chapters 9 and 10.

*Check for shock*

Shock is a depressed condition of the circulatory system. It results in insufficient blood supply to the brain and requires quick intervention as it can threaten life. First aid is virtually powerless in the treatment of haemorrhagic shock for which replenishment of the depleted circulation volume is the only answer.

*Check parts of the body*

The body check should be undertaken in the following order:

head
neck
chest

abdomen
back
external genital organs
arms, hands, fingers
legs, feet, toes

Look for:

internal damage to organs shown by swelling and skin discoloration (i.e. ruptured spleen)
burns
wounds
fractures
dislocations
sprains
strains
contusions

*Check for sudden illness and non-traumatic conditions*

Emergency conditions can, of course, arise from a variety of causes, apart from trauma. In emergencies which do not involve any apparent trauma, the first-aider may proceed to examine the patient for types of illness and non-traumatic problems. When specific problems are not apparent, the first-aider should proceed by reviewing the body systems, making note of the patient's complaints as well as his or her normal and abnormal functioning.

Systems should include:

cardiopulmonary
vascular
urinary
endocrine
digestive and excretory
reproductive
musculoskeletal
skin

**Important signs and symptoms**

A symptom is a departure from normal function in a patient that indicates disease, illness or injury. Pain, dizziness, numbness and nausea are examples.

A sign is a change in normal functioning that can be observed and measured, such as the skin colour, pulse and respiration rates.

The following description of signs and symptoms is composed to help the first-aider to determine the type and severity of the emergency. Specific interpretations are discussed in subsequent chapters according to the classification.

*State of consciousness*

Levels of consciousness may include:

alertness: can communicate and respond to questioning and other stimuli

lethargy: awake, but responding slowly/may be confused about events and surroundings

drowsiness: sleepy, unable to maintain concentration

semiconsciousness: difficulty in communicating and answering questions/little reaction to stimuli

unconsciousness: not communicating/no response to stimuli/no control of movement

Figure 1 shows the 9 levels of response and the common codes used for pupil size and reaction.

*Skin colour*

Pallor or cyanosis (check lips, palms, soles and eyelids of black people).

*Respiration*

Check rate, depth, ease and sound.

*Pulse*

Check rate and *measure* the volume: weak, thready, full, bounding.

*Pupils*

The circulation of blood to the pupils is sensitive to changes in blood pressure and to brain injury, resulting in pressure on the blood vessels. When exposed to light, the pupils normally constrict. If the pupils remain dilated when exposed to light, this usually indicates an insufficient blood supply. Normally the pupils respond in the same manner. If they are unequal, this indicates brain damage or abnormal

**Levels of response**

9. Alert, rational and fully orientated.

8. Automatism. (Appears fully awake, and alert, but gives incorrect information, e.g. name, address, next of kin. Often seen soon after a short period of loss of consciousness.)

7. Drowsy but answers all questions. Mild impairment of orientation.

6. Answers simple questions but confused and irritable, obeys most commands.

5. Answers only Yes or No. Disorientated, restless and confused. Obeys only simplest commands.

4. No obedience to any commands but responds to pain purposefully.

3. No obedience to commands and responds to pain without purpose.

2. Unrousable by any means.

1. Unrousable, no cough reflex and requires artificial respiration.

| **Pupil size** | **Pupil reaction** |
|---|---|
| L = Large | B = Brisk |
| M = Medium | Sl = Sluggish |
| S = Small | F = Fixed |

**Fig. 1** Codes for levels of response, pupil size and pupil reaction.

pressure. Possible causes are injury such as concussion and fractured skull or a cerebrovascular accident.

An overdose of certain drugs may also affect the pupils. Narcotics such as heroin produce pinpoint constriction. Others produce dilated pupils. The first-aider's concern when observation of dilated pupils is made is depressed circulatory function.

The possibility of a glass eye should be considered when examining the eyes of a casualty.

*Pain*

The determination of pain requires a conscious patient as well as systematic questioning and observation by the first-aider, for example:

| | |
|---|---|
| ASK: | Where does it hurt? |
| OBSERVE: | General body area. |
| | Specific anatomical structure. |
| | Extent of painful area. |
| ASK: | What kind of pain? |
| OBSERVE: | Sharp pain. |
| | Dull pain. |
| | Radiating pain. |
| | Slight and tolerable pain. |
| | Severe and intolerable pain. |
| ASK: | When does it hurt? |
| OBSERVE: | All the time. |
| | Intermittently. |
| | Only when touched. |
| | Only when moved. |
| ASK: | How long has it hurt? |
| OBSERVE: | Since injury. |
| | Day/Hours/Minutes. |
| | Gradual onset. |
| | Sudden onset. |

Response to pain varies in individuals: there are different thresholds. If the patient is frightened or hysterical, the pain may feel worse. In some instances of shock, depression or excessive drug or alcohol use, the pain may be masked. Absence of pain is not an indication of severity. Injuries involving nerve damage may disrupt the sensations of pain.

*Ability to move*

Normal movements of the body are dependent upon normal functioning.

Paralysis should be considered as an indication of damage to nerves, the spinal cord or the brain.

Partial movement or painful movement may indicate injury to the musculoskeletal system. Extreme caution must be exercised when examining a patient for ability to move parts of the body. If there is a fracture or injury to the spinal cord, movement can cause severe and serious damage—even quadraplegia.

**The patient should not be asked to demonstrate movement unless the first-aider is sure that the movement will not cause further injury.**

Specific procedures relating to movement are discussed in subsequent chapters.

*Numbness*

A loss of sensation to touch will produce a feeling of numbness in affected parts of the body. The victim may have difficulty in feeling touch or pain induced by the first-aider. This may be because of the disruption of nerve impulses or blood supply.

*Swelling*

A collection of blood, lymph or other body fluid may produce a swelling of body tissues. This is usually more apparent in tissues close to the body surface. Swelling results from injury, infection, allergic reaction and disruption of blood circulation.

*Deformity*

Injury to parts of the body may produce an abnormal positioning or appearance. Dislocated joints and sometimes fractures produce deformity.

Deformity can usually be determined by comparing the injured part with the corresponding uninjured part.

*Discharge from orifices*

Blood, mucus or other fluids coming from orifices without apparent injury are usually an indication of injuries to connecting internal organs or to structures. Note the colour, consistency and amount of the discharge.

*Nausea/vomiting*

Nausea, vomiting, or both can indicate direct involvement of the upper gastrointestinal tract by poisoning or infection. They can also be the result of the body's reaction to stress, trauma or illness. The amount, colour and consistency of the vomited material should be noted.

*Convulsions*

Extremely high body temperature, epilepsy, brain damage and certain toxic agents can cause convulsions.

The first-aider must prevent the patient injuring himself of herself.

The intensity and duration of the convulsions should also be noted.

The signs and symptoms listed in this chapter are major clues which first-aiders can use to determine the type of emergency with which they are dealing.

Their detection depends upon observation, listening and palpation.

Their interpretation and those of more specific signs and symptoms are presented in the relevant chapters.

### Administer appropriate first aid

The selection of appropriate first aid procedures depends upon the interpretation of data. As the examination of a patient begins with an evaluation of vital signs and proceeds from the most serious to the least serious, so should the same priority system be applied to the administration of first aid.

Administration for life-threatening emergencies must precede further examination for less serious conditions. Once the most serious conditions have been cared for, then the first-aider can proceed to examine for the less serious conditions.

Cardiopulmonary arrest and profuse bleeding are given the highest priority. Time is a critical factor here. Poisoning and severe shock also receive high priority.

Next in priority are emergencies which require immediate medical intervention if life is to be maintained. These include coma, heart attack, cerebrovascular accident, extensive burns, heat stroke and surgical emergencies such as ruptured spleen and other internal bleeding. Difficult or complicated childbirth should also be considered as a high priority emergency.

Once the injuries or medical conditions which are a threat to life have been stabilised, the systematic examination should be continued. Only in this way can possible oversight be eliminated.

### Notify authorities and arrange for transport

By definition, first aid is temporary and immediate treatment only. All emergencies must subsequently be referred to hospital or to a medical practitioner. This must be done not only physically to safeguard the patient but legally to safeguard the first-aider.

**When to notify**

The first-aider, while initiating first aid, should also instruct anyone present to call for assistance and to arrange transport to hospital. If the first-aider is alone, it will be necessary for her or him to provide any first aid which is vital to life and then to send for transport.

If the patient's life is not in danger, all appropriate first aid may be carried out before referral is implemented.

In some cases (for example, poisoning) immediate transfer to hospital is the only procedure.

**Whom to notify**

The nature of the emergency and the availability of medical emergency services will determine whom to notify. The first contact point is established through the emergency telephone number. In Great Britain it is 999. In a country where there is no specified number, the nearest hospital, the police or the telephone operator should be contacted.

In the majority of cases, it is best to rely on professional transport. An ambulance is better equipped and has the facilities for getting through traffic quickly. Speed and traffic regulations have to be observed if a private car is used.

When transport is not urgent, it is best to wait to provide the safest and most comfortable form.

The police must be notified if the incident involves violence, a motor accident, or a criminal act.

The fire department should be informed if the emergency involves fire, smoke, threat of fire or explosion, escaping gas or the need for extrication of victims. Special rescue squads are usually available for trapped victims. The first-aider should leave such activity to those who know how to do it if the casualty's life is not in immediate danger. There is a difference between courage and folly.

It is usually not the first-aider's responsibility to inform the casualty's doctor or relatives. If, however, the victim especially requests this, and there is a delay in obtaining medical personnel, the first-aider may have to undertake this task. If so, it is important that the first-aider calmly states who she or he is, what has happened and what is being done. The first-aider should *not* quote either a diagnosis or a prognosis, but should tell the relatives where the patient is being taken.

**Information which will be required**

Certain essential information must be provided when telephoning for help. It is important to think through the sequence to make sure that nothing of importance is omitted. The following should always be given:

- identification: the first-aider's name, telephone number and place from where she or he is calling
- nature of emergency: type of emergency (for example, motorcar accident), number of people involved and the severity of illness or injury
- first aid instructions: what has been done and the assistance and equipment now required
- directions for locating the site of the emergency

The first-aider should speak calmly and clearly. The recipient should be given time to ask any questions and the first-aider should wait until *the other person* hangs up.

## Follow-up care

Procedures which support, supplement and follow the first aid are follow-up care. They may range from general to technical care.

Basically, the first-aider should consider these as follow-up care procedures:

- maintain an open airway and check vital signs
- make the patient as comfortable as possible
- maintain body temperature
- provide reassurance and emotional support
- provide fluids unless contraindicated
- control bystanders
- complete arrangements for referral

The general procedures outlined in this chapter are intended to serve as a framework to be applied to each emergency care situation. They should be borne in mind during study and practice of the remainder of the text.

## CHAPTER 2

# Respiratory Emergencies

Breathing is essential to life. Without the intake of oxygen and the expiration of carbon dioxide by the lungs, and the transport of these gases by the bloodstream, tissue and organ damage or even death can follow. In all cases of unconsciousness, serious injury, or obvious respiratory distress, despite other more obvious injuries the patient may have, the first-aider *must first* check that the airways are clear and that the respirations are adequate enough to maintain life. The pulse should also be checked at the same time.

The first-aider should make the following observations of all patients suffering from respiratory difficulties:

**1.** Respirations—rate and depth of breathing and whether it is regular or irregular.

**2.** Heart rate (either pulse or apex beat)—volume and whether it is regular or irregular.

**3.** Skin colour—temperature and whether it is moist to touch.

If possible these observations should be recorded, but only if this does not interfere with the treatment and care of the patient. The observations may be taken at intervals of 5 to 30 minutes depending on the condition of the patient. The first-aider should loosen any clothing which is tight around the neck or waist. Garments which restrict the chest movement should also be loosened so as to allow full expansion of the lungs. (See Figs 2 and 3.) The first-aider should remain with the patient until help is obtained.

## RESPIRATORY ARREST

Effective respirations will cease if the airways become blocked or severely constricted and urgent treatment is then required. Respiratory

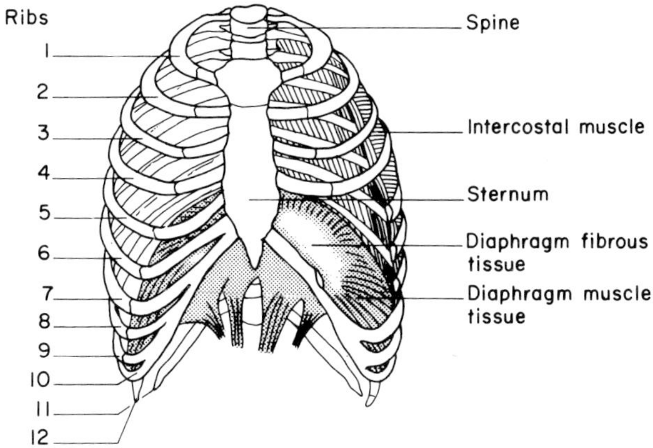


**Fig. 2** The lungs and their protection.

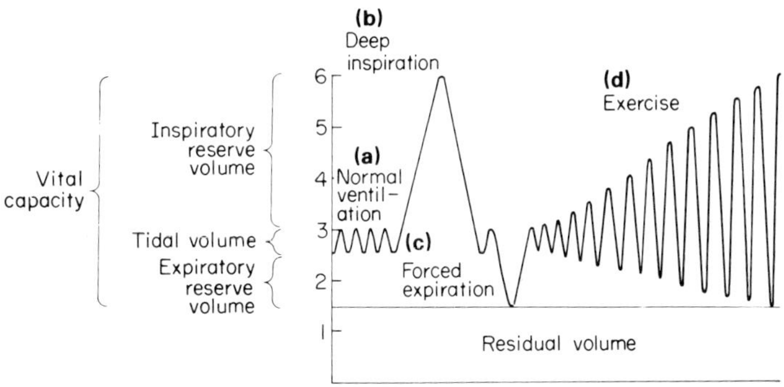


**Fig. 3** Breathing: (a) in normal quiet breathing, there is a short pause between expiration and inspiration; (b and c) voluntary deep breath IN and OUT; and (d) the effect of exercise when breathing is deeper and faster and the pause between breaths disappears.

arrest may occur as the most serious complication of various respiratory diseases, shock or trauma. The present day treatment is to ventilate the patient's lungs artificially. This idea is not new. As far back as the Old Testament, people have been trying to revive the drowned and others whose respirations have ceased, by one means or another. Some methods were of help, such as rolling the victim over a barrel, others,

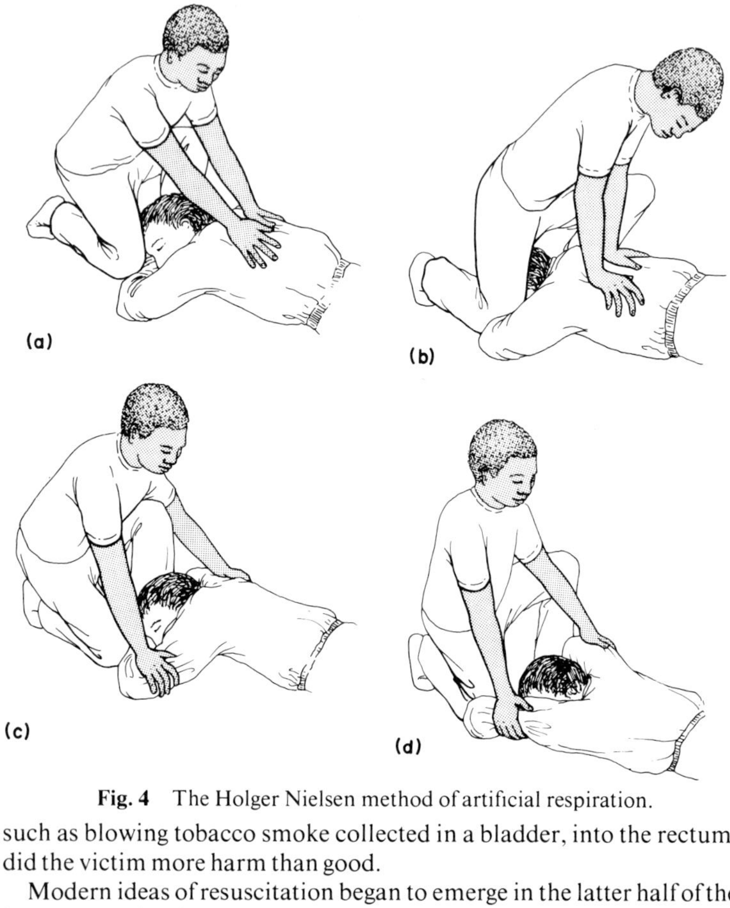


**Fig. 4** The Holger Nielsen method of artificial respiration.

such as blowing tobacco smoke collected in a bladder, into the rectum, did the victim more harm than good.

Modern ideas of resuscitation began to emerge in the latter half of the last century but it was not until Colonel Holger Nielson published a new technique in 1932 (Fig. 4) that effective amounts of air were moved in and out of the lungs. The Holger Nielson method is effective, however, only if the airways are perfectly clear, and it is also a very tiring procedure for the first-aider to perform. That same year, Eve introduced the tilting board method in which the patient was strapped to a stretcher which was then see-sawed. When the head was tilted down, expiration occurred, due to the pressure of the abdominal viscera on the diaphragm, and inspiration occurred in the head upward phase. The disadvantages of this method were that it required special apparatus as well as a trained team.

During the last 15 years, there has been a trend away from these manual methods towards the mouth-to-mouth technique. It has been shown conclusively that this is the only method guaranteed to produce adequate ventilation of the lungs. It can also be performed by a single person without equipment.

**Conditions which may lead to respiratory arrest**

*Severe spasm of the trachea or bronchus.* Causes include: inhalation of a small amount of food or water, smoke, bronchitis, asthma, irritant gases or hiccoughs.

*Obstruction of the airway.* The cause may be the tongue falling back when an unconscious patient is left lying on his or her back; the inhalation of a foreign body or swelling of the tissues due to trauma (insect stings, burns and scalds or the swallowing of corrosives).

*Suffocation* by plastic bags, pillows or other material.

*Compression of the neck*, either by hanging or strangulation.

*Compression of the thoracic cavity.* This can result from a fall of earth, sand or grain in a silo; crushing against a hard object; penetrating wound or the 'flail' chest injury which is commonly seen in road traffic accidents.

*Damage to the nervous system controlling respiration.* This can be caused by:

- electrocution
- poisoning (toxic gases, barbiturates or other overdose of drugs, pesticides)
- muscle spasm (as in tetanus)
- paralysis (as may occur in some diseases such as poliomyelitis, or as the result of injury to the spinal cord)

*The amount of oxygen present in the air is insufficient for the body's needs.* This is usually due to the presence of poisonous gases such as carbon monoxide, the presence of smoke or the changes in atmospheric pressure which occur at high altitudes or during deep sea diving.

*Continuous fitting* (as in status epilepticus).

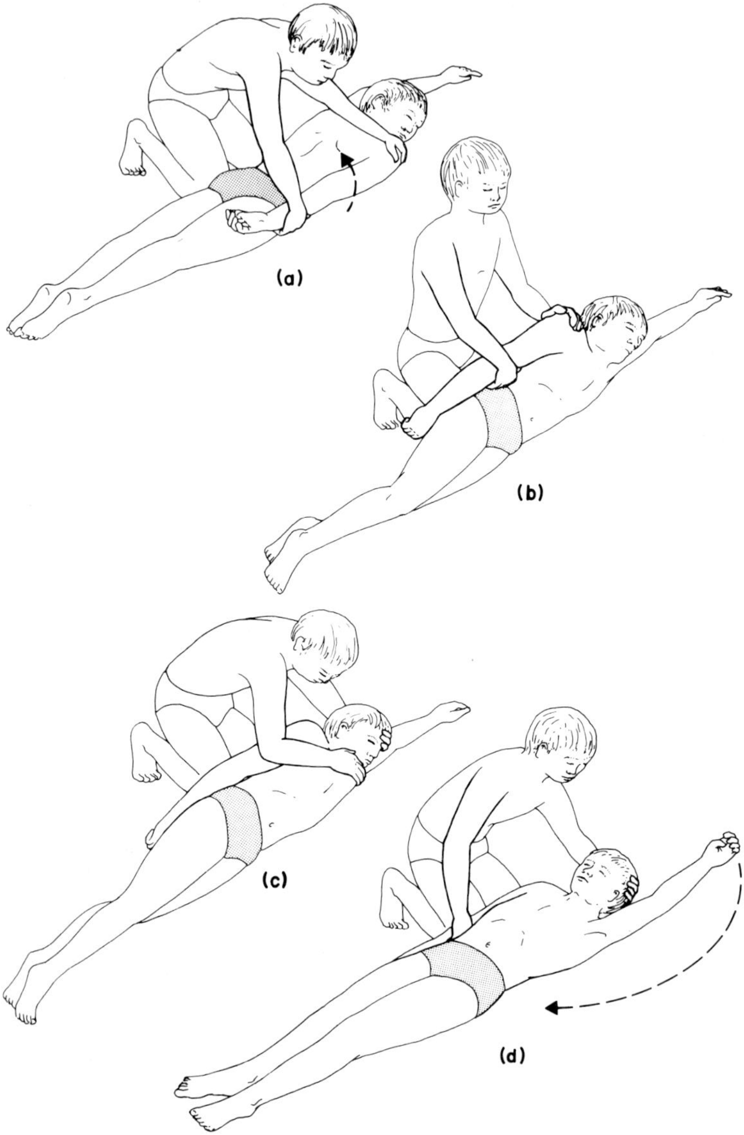


**Fig. 5** Turning a casualty.

SIGNS AND SYMPTOMS

Unconsciousness (in certain cases there may be sudden collapse).

No visible respirations or the patient may gasp intermittently.

Cyanosis of the buccal mucosa and ear lobes.

General pallor or cyanosis.

The carotid pulse is palpable.

Unless artificial respiration is commenced immediatedly, the myocardium will be starved of oxygen and cardiac arrest will follow.

TREATMENT

**1.** If other people are within hearing distance, the first-aider should shout for help.

**2.** Whilst doing **1** the first-aider should ensure that the airway is clear. To do this the patient should be placed flat on his or her back (Fig. 5) with the head turned to one side. If there is a plastic bag over the head or a rope around the neck, these must be cut away before positioning the patient for resuscitation. Vomit or other debris should be scooped out of the mouth with cloth-wrapped fingers (Fig. 6). Usually false teeth should be removed but sometimes whole sets ensure a better seal between the patient's mouth and the first-aider's mouth (see **4**).

**3.** The first-aider should kneel beside the patient's head and ensure that the patient is lying flat. She or he places one hand under the victim's neck, and the other hand under the lower jaw. The head and

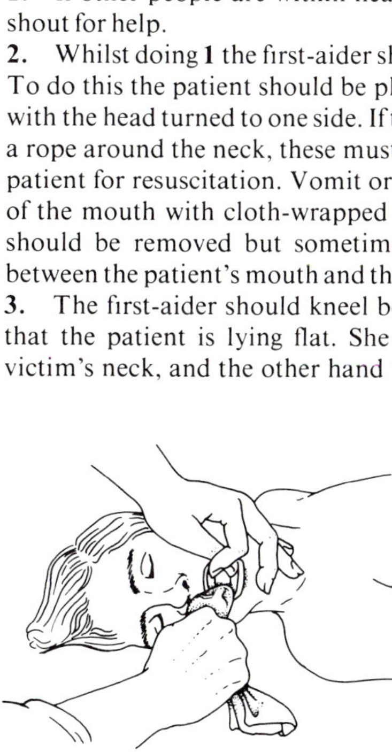

**Fig. 6** Cleaning out the mouth before beginning resuscitation.

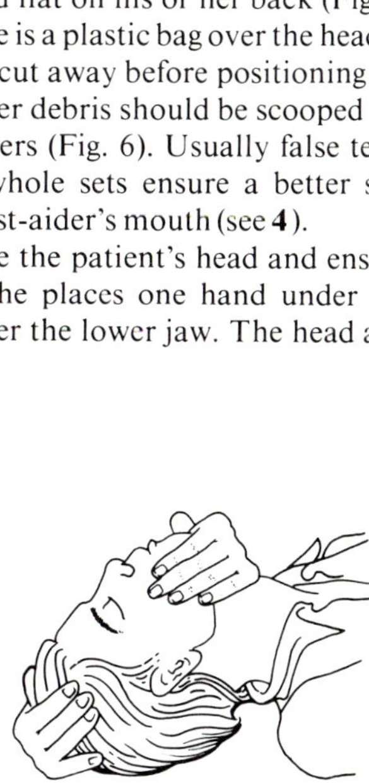

**Fig. 7** Positioning the head.

neck is extended backwards (Fig. 7). This prevents occlusion of the airway by the tongue (Fig. 8).

**4.** After taking a deep breath, the first-aider places her or his mouth over the patient's mouth and forcibly exhales into the patient's lungs (Fig. 9). One hand may continue to support the neck (or preferably a rolled up article of clothing may be used) whilst the other hand pinches the patient's nose. Expiration will occur spontaneously. The first-aider should observe whether or not the patient's chest rises and falls. If it does not, there is either an air leak around the mouth or the airway is blocked. The first-aider should in that case repeat the procedures for clearing the mouth of debris and re-extending the neck, before continuing the procedure. These actions may need to be repeated several times during resuscitation.

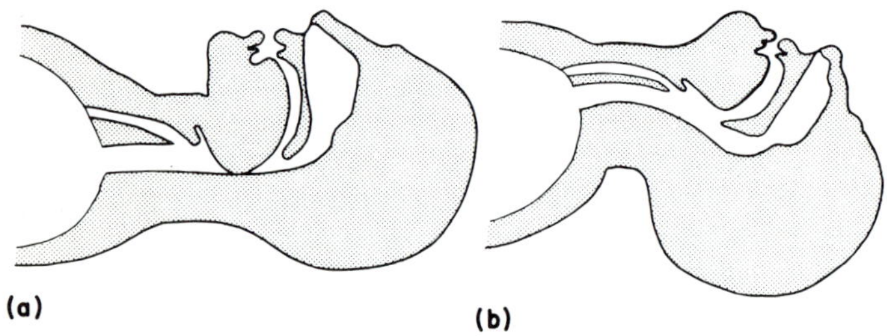


**Fig. 8** Airway (a) blocked by the tongue, and (b) cleared by extending the neck and allowing the free passage of air.

**5.** Whilst carrying out artificial respiration, the first-aider should check the patient's carotid pulse every 2 or 3 minutes to ensure cardiac arrest has not also occurred. Artificial respiration is continued at a rate of 12 to 18 breaths per minute. The procedure may be carried out as mouth-to-nose (Fig. 10) or mouth-to-tracheostomy depending on the patient. In children and infants, both the mouth and nose should be covered by the first-aider's mouth. The younger the child, the more gentle the expiration required to fill the lungs (Fig. 11). Once the chest has been observed to rise, the first-aider should cease to blow and allow expiration to take place spontaneously. Despite the fact that expired breath contains less oxygen (16 per cent as opposed to 21 per cent) and more carbon dioxide (4 per cent as opposed to 0·04 per cent) than atmospheric air, the procedure can be life saving and can be continued until more sophisticated medical equipment arrives (for example, airway, Ambu bag and oxygen) or hospital is reached.

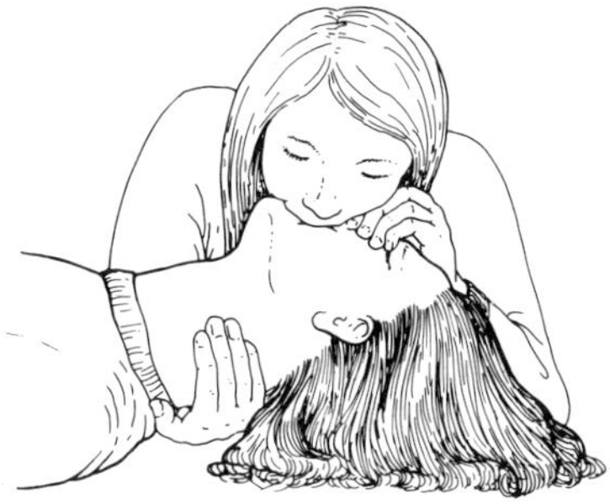

**Fig. 9** Mouth-to-mouth artificial respiration.

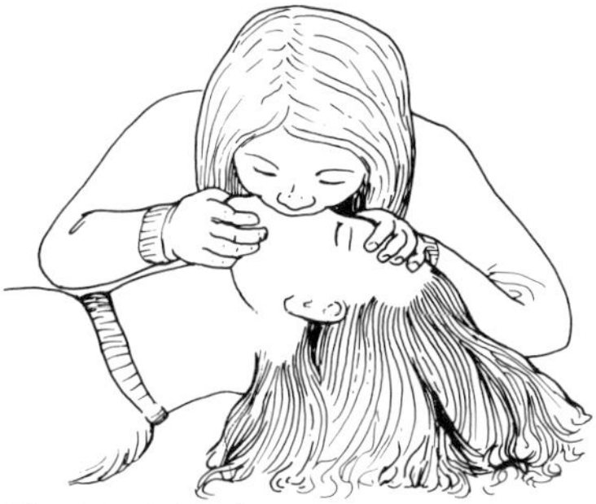

**Fig. 10** Mouth-to-nose artificial respiration.

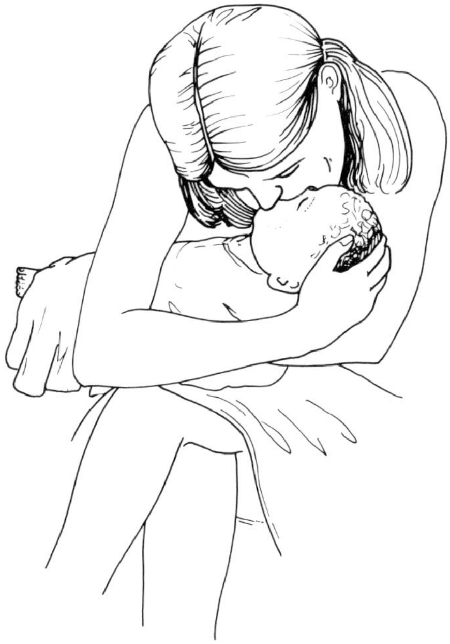

**Fig. 11** Resuscitation of an infant showing the mouth-to-mouth-and-nose position.

Once the patient starts breathing spontaneously (mouth-to-mouth resuscitation may stimulate this) he or she should be placed in the recovery position (Fig. 32). Even if the patient recovers and is apparently unaffected by the respiratory arrest he or she should be taken to hospital as soon as possible, as pulmonary complications may follow.

## INHALATION OF FLUIDS

### Near drowning

Drowning occurs in many varied environments, not just in the sea, lake, river or swimming pool. Drowning can occur in the bath, paddling pool, vats of oil or paint, the sewers and even muddy puddles. Death occurs by asphyxiation due to immersion or submersion in a fluid or liquid medium. This may be the result of epileptic fit, elderly or childhood state, cold, panic, suicide or foul play.

Near drowning occurs when the patient recovers spontaneously or is successfully resuscitated.

### Saline drowning

Sea water contains approximately 3·5 per cent NaCl (salt) whilst blood contains 0·9 per cent NaCl. Therefore, water is drawn out of the circulation by osmosis and this leads to tissue dehydration. As alveolar fluid increases, there is red cell breakdown with resulting acidosis and hypoxia.

### Freshwater drowning

Inhalation of a hypotonic fluid which is rapidly absorbed into the pulmonary capillaries leads to intravascular overload, haemolysis and haemodilution, changes in the alveolar capillary membrane and the composition of pleural surfactant.

### Other fluids

Chemicals such as oil and paint may cause severe damage to the tissues and mucosal linings.

In all cases of drowning artificial respiration must be commenced at once and continued either until the patient recovers or a doctor declares the patient dead. When patients recover spontaneously the first-aider should then treat them for shock. All cases of near drowning should be examined by a doctor as pulmonary complications nearly always follow. The first-aider, therefore, should arrange for the victim to be transferred to hospital as soon as possible.

## INHALATION OF A FOREIGN BODY

Inhalation of a foreign body is not uncommon, but most people's cough reflex is strong enough for the foreign body to be exhaled spontaneously. Commonly inhaled foreign bodies are: particles of food, fish and meat bones, small coins and beads.

### SIGNS AND SYMPTOMS

The patient chokes and tries to cough and then makes desperate attempts at inhalation. He or she becomes cyanosed, and the head and neck appear congested.

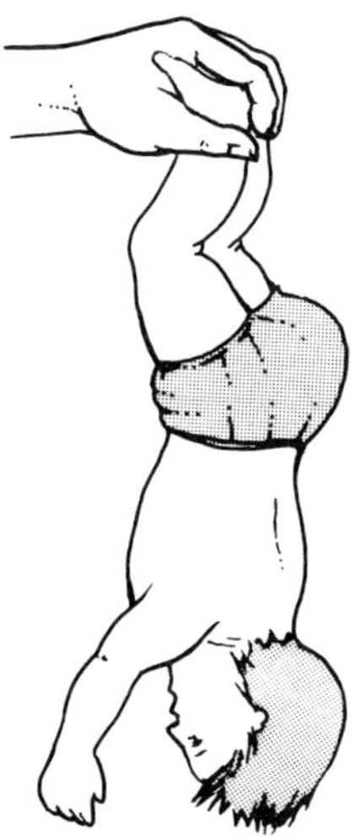

**Fig. 12** Removal of an inhaled foreign body in an infant.

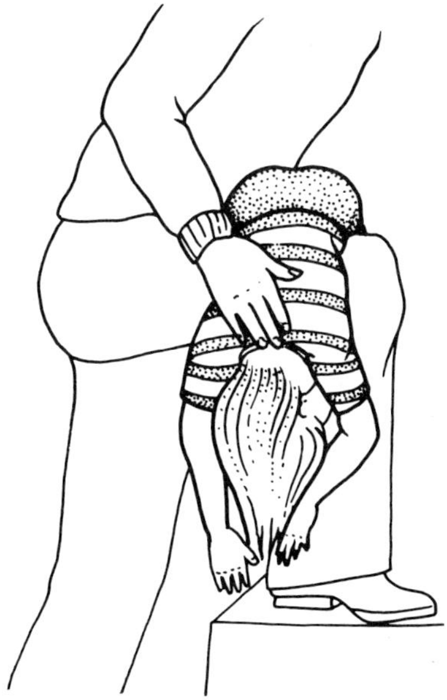

**Fig. 13** Removal of an inhaled foreign body in a child.

TREATMENT

The first-aider should **not** attempt to remove the foreign body with the fingers as this may only push it further down the airway. The following procedure(s) should be carried out immediately:

BABIES AND INFANTS—the first-aider should hold the baby upside down by the feet and smack firmly between the shoulder blades (Fig. 12).

CHILDREN—the first-aider should lie the child face down over her or his knee or arm and smack the child sharply between the shoulder blades (Fig. 13).

ADULTS—there are two methods available and either may be used, depending on the circumstances.

*Method a* The patient should be grasped around the thorax (under the sternum) by the first-aider standing behind and given a short, sharp bear-hug (Fig. 14).

*Method b* The patient is told to lean over the back of a chair and the first-aider then bangs him or her sharply 3 or 4 times between the shoulder blades (Fig. 15).

The foreign body should dislodge and be coughed out. In cases where very soft food, drink, blood or vomit is inhaled, the patient should be placed in the recovery position (Fig. 32) and debris cleared from the mouth. If breathing has ceased, then artificial respiration should be commenced.

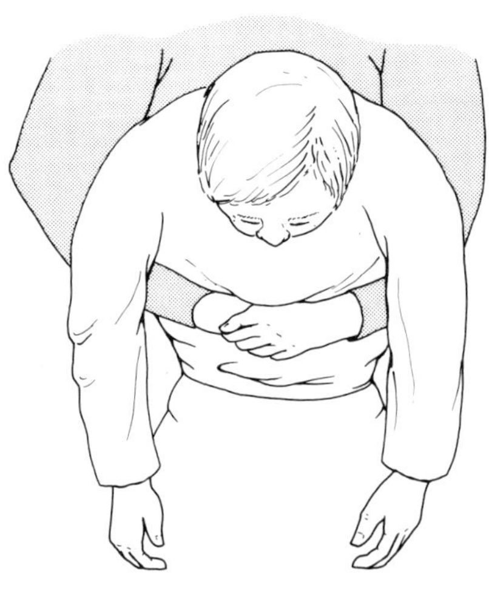

**Fig. 14** Procedure for dislodging aspirated chunk of food, showing the important positioning of the first-aider's hands under the sternum.

**Note:** This method should only be used following practical instruction and practice.

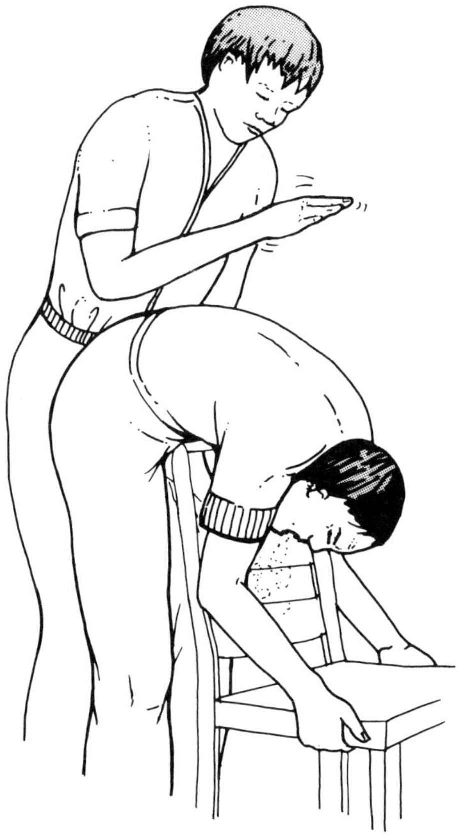

**Fig. 15** Removal of an inhaled foreign body in an adult.

In cases of a hard object not being exhaled, it sometimes lodges in the entrance to one bronchus, allowing air to enter the other lung. Much of the breathing difficulties experienced in these cases is due to spasm of the trachea and bronchi. The first-aider should reassure and calm the patient. The patient will probably feel most comfortable in the sitting position. The first-aider should check the pulse and respirations every 15 minutes. Transfer to hospital for treatment must be arranged immediately.

## INHALATION OF TOXIC GASES

The most common toxic gas to be inhaled is carbon monoxide (see also pages 164–5). Though the mortality rate from carbon monoxide poisoning has diminished, because of the reduced use of 'town gas', natural gas (and others), may be harmful in a closed space simply because they displace the amount of oxygen available. The first-aider may also encounter carbon monoxide poisoning due to inhalation of vehicle exhaust fumes. These cases are often attempted suicides.

### SIGNS AND SYMPTOMS

The smell of the gas is usually evident. However, if the gas has seeped through a layer of earth there may be no smell. The victim may be disorientated or unconscious depending on the degree of hypoxia. The pulse may be irregular due to cardiac arrhythmias. Severe hypotension and cardiac failure are often features. In carbon monoxide poisoning the gas combines strongly with haemoglobin to form carboxyhaemoglobin, and this makes the patient's skin appear pale pink in colour instead of cyanosed as occurs normally in hypoxia; patchy erythema and bullae may also develop.

### TREATMENT

The first action of the first-aider is to remove the patient from the source of gas and preferably out of doors. Artificial respiration should be given if necessary. The first-aider should observe the casualty's skin colour, pulse and respiration rates every 5 to 10 minutes. The patient should be immediately taken to hospital, resuscitative measures being maintained during the journey if necessary.

## PULMONARY EMBOLISM

Pulmonary embolism is the blockage of one or more of the pulmonary arteries and arterioles. The embolus may be a piece (or pieces) of clot which has broken off a thrombosis elsewhere in the body, or a fat embolism from a fractured limb. The severity of the resulting signs and symptoms depends on the size of the embolus (or emboli).

### SIGNS AND SYMPTOMS

In severe cases where the embolus is large the patient will collapse suddenly, suffering from respiratory and cardiac arrests.

In cases of a smaller embolus, the patient will complain of a 'tight' chest pain, similar to that of myocardial infarction but which does not (usually) radiate to the neck or arms. The patient may expectorate blood and appear dyspnoeic. He or she may also appear shocked and the skin cyanosed or pallid.

When the patient has suffered multiple small emboli the clinical features are less easy to distinguish. The patient may complain of mild pain over those areas of lung which have been infarcted. Dyspnoea and haemoptysis may also be features.

### TREATMENT

In cases of sudden collapse resuscitative procedures should be applied whilst the patient is quickly transferred to hospital.

Where a smaller embolus is suspected the patient should lie flat and move as little as possible. This is to prevent the dislodgement of further emboli. The first-aider should check for signs and symptoms of a deep-vein thrombosis in order to help distinguish the cause of pain from that of myocardial infarction.

The most common site of a deep-vein thrombosis is the calf. The affected area may appear red and swollen and will usually be warmer to touch than the surrounding skin. The patient may also complain that the affected area is painful.

The casualty who has a fractured limb and complains of chest pain may also be suffering from a pulmonary embolus due to fat escaping into the bloodstream from the bone's central canal. The first-aider should treat the patient for shock and observe the pulse and respiration rates and skin colour every 5 to 10 minutes. If possible, any blood expectorated should be collected in a suitable receptacle for later inspection by a doctor. The patient should be transported to hospital as quickly and as smoothly as possible.

## SPONTANEOUS PNEUMOTHORAX

When part of the lung tissue is torn, air escapes from the lung into the pleural cavity. As pressure in the pleural cavity is normally lower than

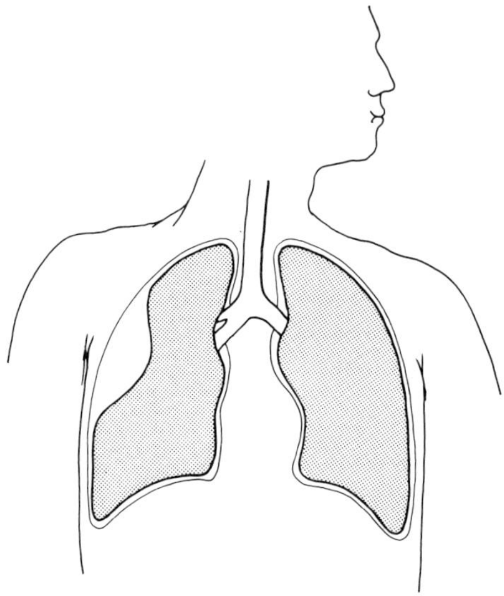

**Fig. 16** A pneumothorax showing a collapsed lung.

that of the lung, the presence of air causes a rise in pressure and the lung collapses (Fig. 16).

SIGNS AND SYMPTOMS

The patient often complains of severe pain on the affected side of the chest and there is sudden onset of breathlessness. If a large portion of the lung is collapsed, the patient may become hypoxic and cyanosed, and may also suffer shock.

TREATMENT

The first-aider should place the patient in a comfortable resting position which allows maximum expansion of the unaffected lung. Observe the patient's pulse and respirations at regular intervals. Transport to hospital should be arranged as quickly as possible.

COMPLICATIONS

If the pneumothorax is of the tension type in which a 'flap' valve allows air to pass from the lung into the pleural cavity but not out again, surgical emphysema may develop. This may be recognised by the skin appearing puffy and crackling when touched. This is due to the presence of subcutaneous air. The patient should be transferred to hospital as a matter of urgency, as very high pressure in the pleural cavity may lead to further complications such as mediastinal shift.

## ASTHMA

Asthma is a disease which may be episodic or chronic.

### SIGNS AND SYMPTOMS

Asthma is characterised by paroxysms of dyspnoea accompanied by wheezing resulting from temporary narrowing of the bronchi by muscle spasms, mucosal oedema or viscid secretions. This bronchial narrowing prevents adequate ventilation of the lungs. It also raises the resistance to air flow in the bronchi, especially during expiration. This causes air to be trapped in the lungs. The patient often suffers prolonged spells of coughing in an effort to clear the secretions. Asthmatics are usually tense, anxious people who became severely distressed during an attack.

### TREATMENT

The first-aider is most likely to be involved in caring for acute attacks of asthma. In mild attacks the asthmatic patient will require only reassurance and perhaps help in using inhalers such as salbutamol. In more severe cases, the first-aider should place the patient in a comfortable sitting position, to allow full lung expansion, and should be given plenty of fresh air. Calm assurance from the first-aider that the patient will soon be able to breathe again will do much to help. However frightened and overanxious an asthmatic patient may seem, neither sedation nor alcohol should be given as this will reduce the respiratory drive so desperately needed. If the patient has bronchodilators, such as aminophylline or salbutamol, they should be given as directed. Sips of water may also be given. The first-aider should provide a suitable receptacle as a sputum pot (an old yoghurt carton for instance) as thick mucoid secretions will be expectorated.

When the asthma attack is severe or prolonged, a doctor should be called urgently or the patient taken to hospital.

## ACUTE CHEST INFECTIONS

The first-aider may occasionally be called upon to deal with patients suffering from acute chest infections as mild signs and symptoms sometimes become severe either suddenly or over a short period of time. Often the patient will have had no other indication than having felt 'off colour' for a day or so previously.

The group of infections includes those causing pneumonia, acute bronchitis, acute exacerbations of chronic bronchitis and emphysema.

### SIGNS AND SYMPTOMS

The patient appears and feels generally unwell. The temperature is usually raised and the skin dry and hot. Cyanosis and pallor may be features. The patient will be dyspnoeic and may expectorate thick purulent sputum. In cases of pneumonia, the sputum may appear rust-coloured. The patient may complain of generalised chest pain.

### TREATMENT

Dyspnoeic patients should be made as comfortable as possible in a semirecumbent position propped up with pillows so arranged as to allow maximum chest expansion. The temperature should be taken if a thermometer is available, and pulse and respiration rates checked. Sputum should be saved for inspection by a doctor. If the patient has previously been supplied with a home oxygen cylinder, oxygen may be given as necessary. If the patient has chronic bronchitis the oxygen should be given in a low concentration (24 per cent), and the dose previously ordered by the doctor should not be exceeded. A high concentration of oxygen administered to chronic bronchitis will cause carbon dioxide retention and respiratory failure.

A steam inhalation may be given, provided extreme caution is exercised. A bowl or jug of steaming water should be placed on a table in front of the patient and a towel placed over the patient's head as he or she leans over the bowl. The first-aider must hold the bowl to prevent spillage. The patient should inhale the steam as deeply as possible. (Steam inhalations should *never* be given to children or confused or elderly patients who may tip the inhalation over and scald themselves.) Inhalations will loosen thick sputum and ease expectoration.

Patients with chest infections often become dehydrated so plenty of fluids should be encouraged. The patient's general practitioner should be asked to visit as soon as possible.

## HYPERVENTILATION

Hyperventilation is a condition often associated with hysteria.

### SIGNS AND SYMPTOMS

The hyperventilated patient has a very high respiratory rate and overventilates, causing an abnormally low level of carbon dioxide in the bloodstream. This may lead to alkalosis and the patient may experience painful cramps in the limbs and tingling of the hands and feet (tetany).

### TREATMENT

The first-aider must be calm and reassuring. The patient should be made to re-breathe his or her own air (for example, from a brown *paper* bag). This will ensure that the patient inhales a high level of carbon dioxide and the alkalosis is thus corrected. The tingling in the hands and feet should also disappear. If the patient starts to overbreathe again the symptoms will reappear and the treatment should be repeated. Usually this will not happen more than once, as the patient will be impressed by the demonstration of the origin of his or her symptoms. He or she should be examined by a doctor as soon as possible as the hysteria may require treatment.

## CHEST INJURIES

Wounds to the chest may take on various forms—from stab wounds to the impact of heavy industrial machinery or a steering wheel.

### Simple penetrating wounds

Simple penetrating wounds are usually made by a knife or bullet.

#### TREATMENT

If the weapon is still in situ, the first-aider should not attempt to remove it as this may only increase haemorrhage. After checking that the patient is not in need of any resuscitative measures and that the airway is clear, the first-aider should deal with the wound.

The usual complications of this type of wound are pneumothorax and haemothorax caused by the entry of air and blood into the pleural cavity via the wound. The aim of the first-aider in dressing the wound is to minimise these two complications. Air entry via the wound is often audible; 'sucking' as the patient breathes. The first-aider should dress the wound so that it is as air-tight as possible. A dry dressing covered by a piece of polythene (for example, a plastic bag) firmly taped down around the edges is best. A firm dressing will also help to control haemorrhage.

The first-aider should check both for entry and exit points of the weapon or bullet, as both will require dressing.

The patient should be treated for shock, and pulse, respirations and skin colour observations made at quarter hourly intervals. No food or drink should be given. The patient should be transferred to hospital as quickly as possible for treatment.

## Crushed chest injuries

### Simple fracture of the ribs

One or more ribs broken in one place only is a simple fracture. The patient will complain of localised pain. This is made worse by deep breathing, coughing or movement. The patient will often lean to the affected site and support the injured area with his or her hand.

#### TREATMENT

The first-aider should dress any surface injuries. The arm on the injured side (or both arms if necessary) should be strapped to the patient's chest or put in a sling to immobilise it (Figs 17 and 18). Since removing the clothes may cause undue pain and exposure, the bandage should be applied over the clothing. The bandage should be tightened during expiration. It should not be overtight as the end of a fractured rib can puncture a lung. The patient should be seated in as comfortable a position as possible. The first-aider should, if necessary, treat for shock. Obervations of the pulse, respiration rate and skin colour should be made at regular intervals, depending on the patient's condition. He or she should be taken to hospital as soon as possible.

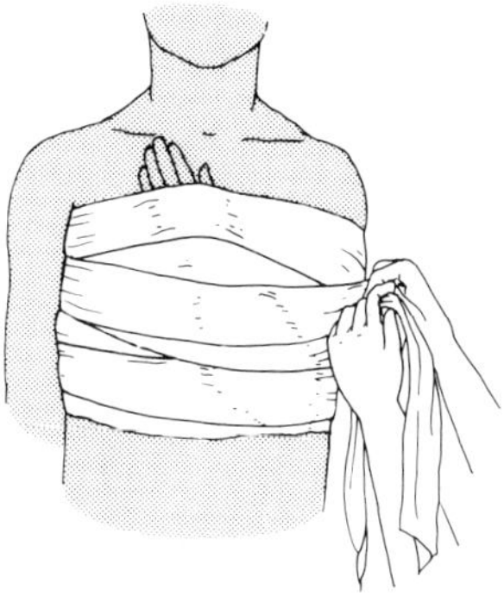

**Fig. 17** Bandaging to immobilise fractured ribs.

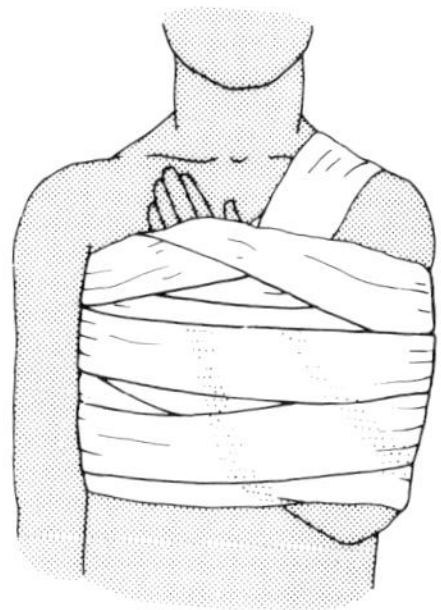

**Fig. 18** Strapping the patient's arm to his chest to immobilise a flail chest.

COMPLICATIONS

Occasionally the end of a fractured rib will puncture the lung. In such cases a degree of pneumothorax or haemothorax occurs. The patient should be treated (as described on page 90) for these conditions and transferred to hospital immediately.

## Flail (stove in) chest

In cases of flail chest more than one rib is fractured, and each rib broken in two or more places (Fig. 19). The segment of the chest wall between these breaks will collapse each time the patient attempts to breathe. The 'flail' or loose segment will move paradoxically to the rest of the thoracic cage when the patient tries to breathe. The underlying lung and mediastinal structures are usually seriously damaged; surgical emphysema, haemothorax and pneumothorax are common complications.

SIGNS AND SYMPTOMS

The patient will complain of severe pain and the first-aider will observe that the chest does not rise properly despite the patient's most desperate efforts to breathe deeply. He or she will appear severely shocked and may cough up fresh blood.

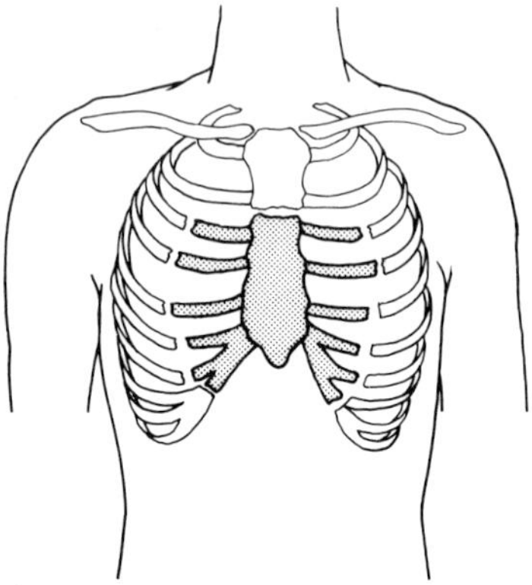

**Fig. 19** Flail chest.

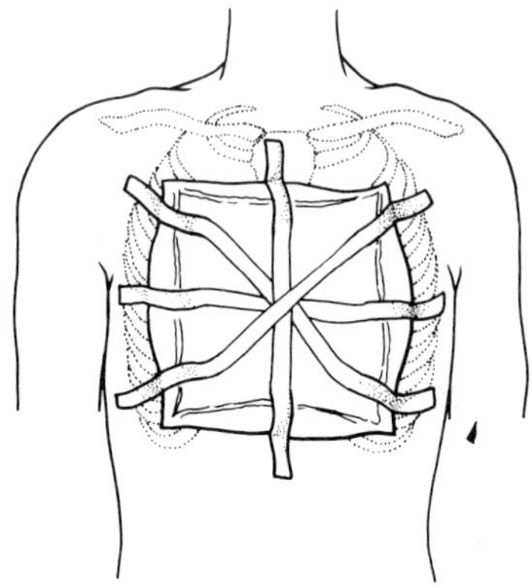

**Fig. 20** Immobilisation of a flail chest using a small pillow and strapping.

TREATMENT

If breathing is inadequate and the patient cyanosed, then mouth-to-mouth artificial respiration must be given until other ventilating equipment arrives or until the patient is transferred to hospital for positive pressure ventilation.

If possible the first-aider should splint the chest, either by strapping a firm object such as a small cushion over the flail portion of the chest (Fig. 20) or by strapping the patient's arms to the chest (Figs 17 and 18). This splinting will enable the patient to breathe on his or her own more easily.

The patient should be positioned according to the injuries—if the injury is to the front of the chest and he or she is conscious, then a semirecumbent position is best. Otherwise the patient should lie with his or her head and shoulders raised and his or her body inclined towards the injured side. The patient should be supported in this position by pillows or a folded blanket placed lengthways along his or her back.

The first-aider should treat the patient for shock and observe the skin colour, pulse and respiration rates every 5 to 10 minutes.

This is a serious respiratory emergency for which the only treatment is positive pressure ventilation even if the patient does not require immediate resuscitative measures. Immediate transportation to hospital should be arranged.

## ANAPHYLACTIC SHOCK

Anaphylactic shock occurs as an extreme allergic reaction. The patient who has become sensitised to a substance by previous contact with it, reacts violently to another dose or contact.

Methods and some examples of substances causing such reactions may be:

injected—antibiotics
ingested—foods, such as shell fish or oral antibiotics
insect stings 'injected'—bee, wasp or hornet
inhaled—pollens

### SIGNS AND SYMPTOMS

At first the patient may experience flushing, itching or burning sensations especially on the face and upper chest. Hives may spread over large areas of the body. Oedema of the face and tongue may quickly develop and the lips may become rapidly cyanosed. Within a short time, the patient may become dyspnoeic, complain of pain in the chest, cough and wheeze. The pulse will become weak, and the patient will feel dizzy and may collapse suddenly with respiratory or cardiac arrest.

### TREATMENT

Resuscitation procedures as necessary should be commenced at once. If they are not needed, the first-aider should put the patient in the recovery position and skin colour, pulse and respiration rates should be observed every 5 to 10 minutes. Nothing should be given by mouth. Transportation to hospital should be arranged urgently in order that drugs may be given to counteract the effects of the allergy.

CHAPTER 3

# Cardiac Emergencies

As respiration is essential to life, so is the ability of the heart to circulate blood around the body, transporting oxygen and nutrients to the tissues and removing carbon dioxide and other waste products of metabolism (Fig. 21). Impairment or total failure of this pumping action leads to disablement or death of the individual.

The first-aider should make the same observations of patients suffering from cardiac emergencies as those listed for respiratory emergencies since the two systems are closely allied. Some mention must be made at this point about the first-aider's observation of heart

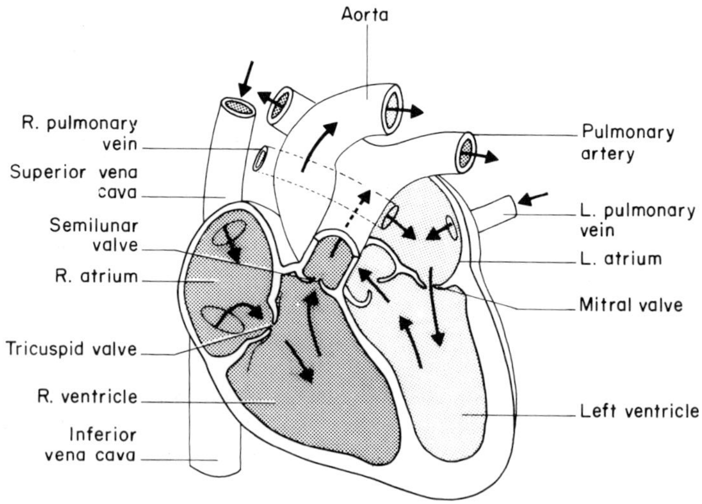


**Fig. 21** The circulation of the blood in the heart.

rate. In cardiac and respiratory conditions the peripheral circulation is very often shut down, and the peripheral pulses such as the radial pulse are not palpable; this may lead to a mis-diagnosis of cardiac arrest. It is therefore necessary to feel for the pulses nearer to the central circulation. The three methods of doing this are:

**1** Palpating the carotid pulse in the neck. This is easily found by turning the patient's head a little to the side and moving the fingers directly downwards from the ear lobe (Fig. 22).

**2** Palpating the femoral pulse in the groin (Fig. 23).

**3** Listening to the apex beat of the heart by placing an ear on the patient's chest below the left nipple. Without the aid of a stethoscope this last method is less reliable than the other two.

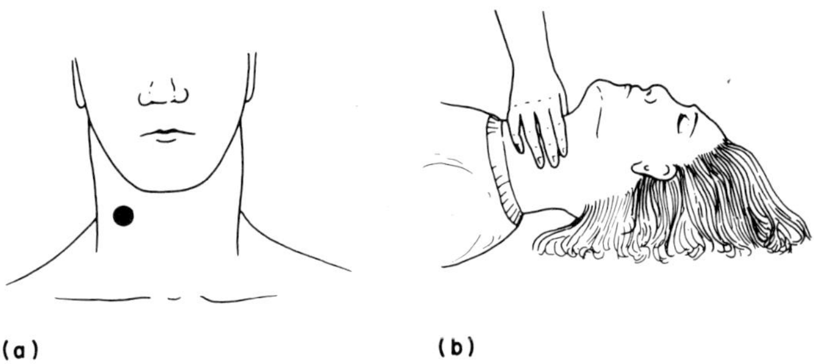

**Fig. 22** The position (a) and the palpation (b) of the carotid pulse.

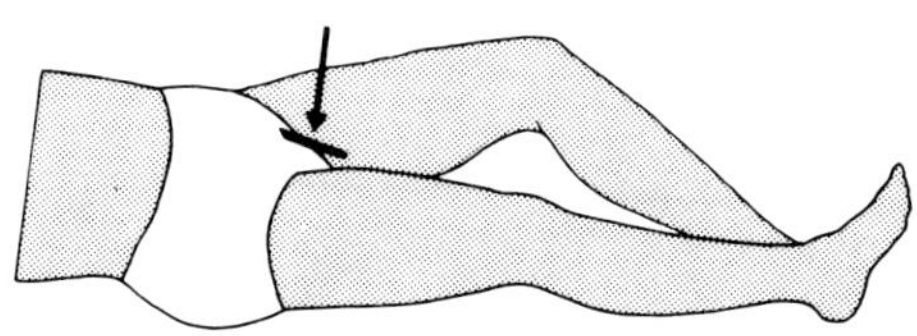

**Fig. 23** Position of the femoral pulse.

## CARDIAC ARREST

When the heart stops beating or is beating in such a manner that little or no blood is circulating (as in ventricular fibrillation) then the patient may be said to be clinically dead, and biological death will follow about 3 minutes later.

Methods of reviving patients whose hearts have stopped are relatively modern, although experiments with electrical shocks and their effects on the heart (defibrillation as we know it) date from the 17th century. Cardiac massage dates from the middle of the last century. In 1858, James Balassa of Budapest is recorded as having successfully carried out a form of external cardiac massage on a girl suffering from tuberculosis laryngitis.

The scientific study of cardiac compression dates from 1874, with the experimental work of Professor Schiff. He demonstrated that sudden death in dogs submitted to chloroform was usually associated with ventricular fibrillation rather than asystole, and that if the chest was opened, the heart could be rhythmically compressed and the heart beat restored. Similar experiments continued over the years with varying success, internal cardiac compression via the abdominal route being the most popular.

It was not until 1960 in the United States that external cardiac massage (ECM) was reintroduced. Kouwenhoven and his colleagues at Johns Hopkins Hospital, Baltimore, Maryland, demonstrated that closed cardiac compression could, in many cases, be effectively applied by people who had no medical background—only a training in that one technique. This proved to be a turning point in the history of resuscitation.

### Conditions which may lead to cardiac arrest

Conditions which may lead to cardiac arrest includes all those which may lead to respiratory arrest, plus

Myocardial infarction
Failure of the cardiac conducting mechanism
Cardiogenic shock

#### SIGNS AND SYMPTOMS

Unconsciousness—often occurring as a sudden collapse. No palpable pulses; (feel for either the carotid or femoral pulse).
Apnoea.
Dilating pupils, or (by 40 seconds post-collapse) dilated pupils.
Grey or white or cyanosed (blue) skin.

The patient is, in effect, clinically dead. Unless effective ventilation and circulation are started within 3 minutes biological death will follow.

If other people are within hearing, the first-aider should shout for help while preparing to treat the patient.

TREATMENT

Lay the patient flat on a firm hard surface and with a closed fist give a sharp bang on the lower third of the sternum (Fig. 24). This may be enough to restart the heart beat without further action. This procedure should only be used on adults.

Check the patient's pulses again; if they are still absent then clear the airway prior to commencing external cardiac massage and artificial respiration at a ratio of 1 breath to every 6 compressions. The patient's lungs should be inflated before external cardiac massage is commenced.

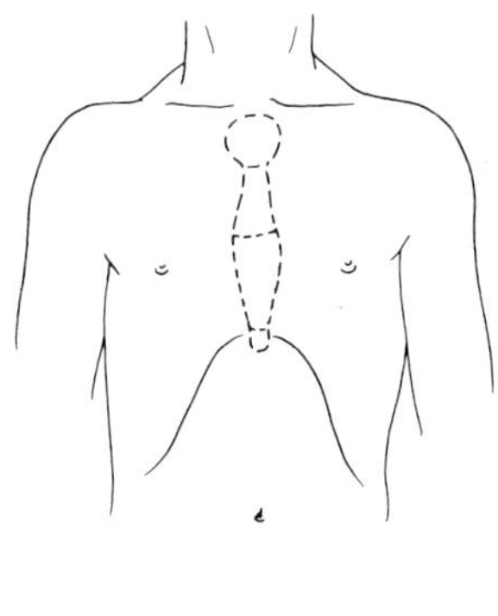

**Fig. 24** The position of the sternum showing the area (shaded) to be compressed.

## External cardiac massage (ECM)

For massage to be effective, the patient must be lying on a firm flat surface. The principle of ECM is to compress the heart between the sternum and the spine, thus literally squeezing blood out of it (Fig. 25). The first-aider should kneel as close as possible to the patient's side, at right angles to him or her and alongside the thorax. The lower third of the sternum should be pressed down sharply with the heels of the hands working from the shoulders (Fig. 26). The arms should not bend at the elbows. The rate of compressions should be 70–80 per minute (the normal pulse rate). The first-aider should check the carotid pulse every few minutes to see if the patient's heart beat has restarted. The pupils

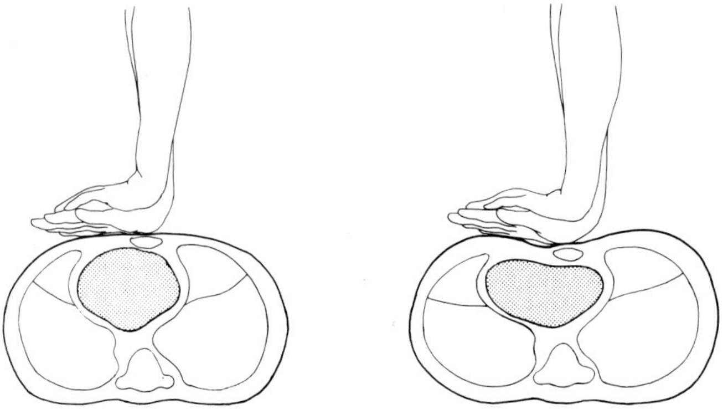

**Fig. 25** Compression of the heart between the sternum and the spine.

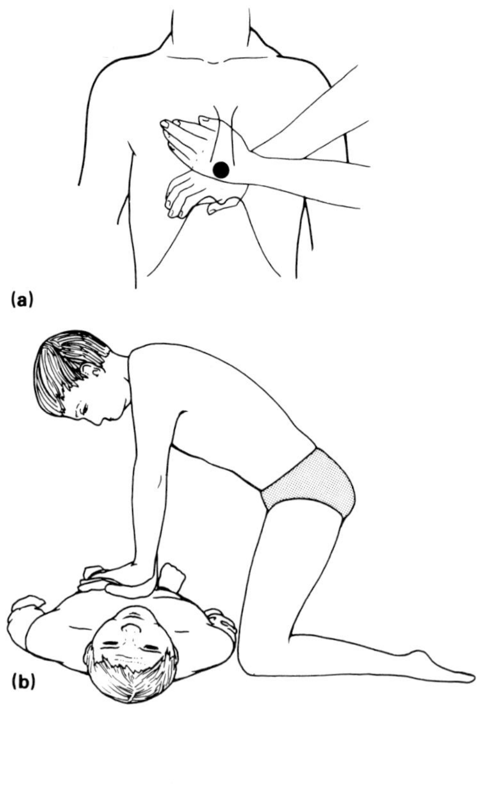


**Fig. 26** External cardiac massage showing the position of (a) the heels of the hands on the lower third of the sternum and (b) the operator with straight arms working from the shoulders.

should also be checked every few minutes—if the first-aider is administering effective ventilation and massage they will begin to constrict.

It is possible for one person to carry out both the ECM and artificial ventilation effectively but it is very tiring, and if two first-aiders are available, once an ambulance has been called, they should work together.

One first-aider should care for the airway and ventilation and the other one perform ECM (Fig. 27). The first-aider caring for the airway should check the carotid pulse at regular intervals of 2 to 3 minutes, whilst the massager stops for a few seconds. There should also be a pause after every sixth massage to allow ventilation. The first-aider should check that the patient's chest is inflating. The size of the pupils can be easily checked by the first-aider caring for the airway.

Effective cardiac massage and ventilation can be continued by two people for a considerable length of time if they change roles every few minutes. It may be necessary to continue until a hospital is reached and the staff there take over. If the patient's pulse recommences, the first-aider should check whether respiration has also recommenced. It may be necessary to continue artificial ventilation without the massage. If the patient has recovered both facilities, then he or she should be placed in the recovery position (Fig. 32). The first-aider should in both cases monitor the pulse rate at 2 to 3 minute intervals and in the latter case also observe the respirations. Even if the patient recovers consciousness and appears to be all right, he or she should still be taken

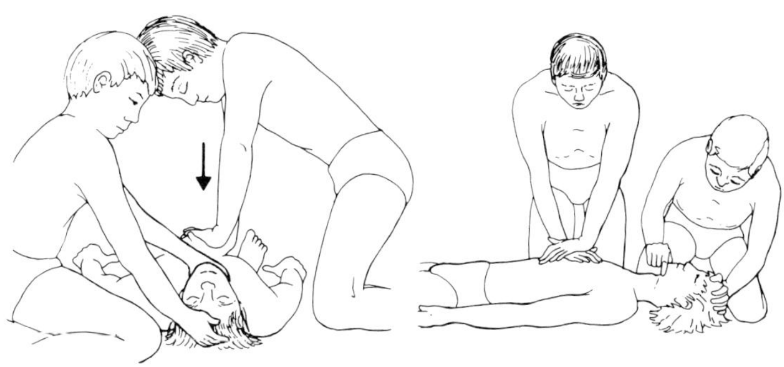

**Fig. 27** External cardiac massage with two operators showing alternative positions.

to hospital as an emergency, as there may be pulmonary and cardiac complications; or, if effective ventilation and massage has not been started early enough, brain and kidney damage.

**ECM for children and babies**

The younger the child, the less pressure the first-aider should apply to the lower third of the sternum. In children, adequate pressure can be applied using the heel of only one hand (Fig. 28) and in babies two fingers are adequate (Fig. 29). The initial bang on the chest given to adults should **never** be administered to children or babies.

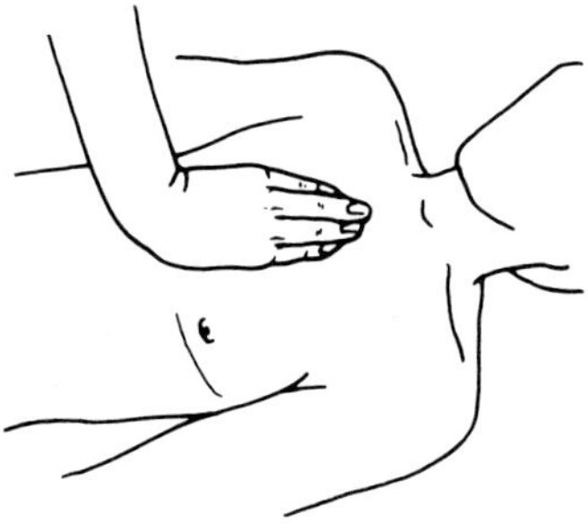

**Fig. 28** External cardiac massage on a child.

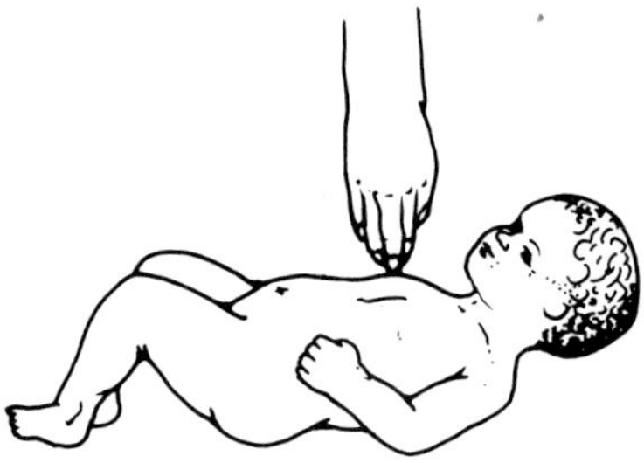

**Fig. 29** External cardiac massage on a baby.

**Other complications of cardiopulmonary resuscitation**

In her or his efforts to resuscitate the patient, the first-aider may induce the following complications:

fractured ribs (including flail chest)
fractured sternum
pneumothorax due to puncture of the lung by a fractured rib
lacerations and contusions of the lungs, heart, liver and spleen

These complications are avoidable if the procedure is carried out correctly. The possibility of breaking the ribs can be avoided if the fingers are kept away from the chest wall and pressure applied only via the heels of the hands, straight downwards from the shoulders. Pressure must also be applied only to the lower third of the sternum and never to the xiphoid sternum or elsewhere on the chest.

**Who should not be resuscitated?**

Most people who collapse suddenly and inexplicably should be resuscitated unless it is known for certain that clinical death occurred more than 5 minutes previously. Cardiac arrest occurring as part of natural death due to old age or the terminal stages of a chronic disease such as cancer, should not be reversed by resuscitation.

It can be a difficult decision for the first-aider to make, but it helps if it is known the exact time collapse occurred and also whether the heart stopped beating at the same time as respiration ceased. If the heart continued to beat for 2 or 3 minutes after respiratory arrest, oxygen would still have been circulating in the body and the onset of brain damage delayed.

If, on the other hand, the first-aider knows that the brain has been without oxygen for more than 5 or 6 minutes, cardiopulmonary resuscitation should not be attempted. Even if 'successful', and the respirations and heart beat are restarted, the victim will have suffered severe brain damage and be doomed to a vegetable-like existence.

## CARDIAC DISORDERS

### Angina

When the coronary arteries become thrombosed, the blood supply to the myocardium is reduced, causing ischaemia and pain.

SIGNS AND SYMPTOMS

The patient complains of pain like a tight band around the chest which may radiate down one or both arms. He or she may appear dyspnoeic. Angina is usually precipitated by exercise but may also be brought on by anxiety or by eating a heavy meal.

TREATMENT

The first-aider should sit the patient in a comfortable position. If the patient has suffered previously from angina and carries glycerine trinitrate pills (TNT), the first-aider should place one under his or her tongue. Pulse and respiration rates should be taken and noted. Pain usually passes off within a few minutes. If it is the first time the patient has experienced such pain, he or she should be taken at once to a doctor or to a hospital as myocardial infarction should always be suspected in these instances. The same applies if the pain is unrelieved by TNT and rest.

## Myocardial infarction (heart attack)

When complete blockage of a coronary artery occurs, the blood supply to that area of myocardium ceases and tissue death ensues.

SIGNS AND SYMPTOMS

The patient complains of a tight gripping pain like a band around the chest which radiates down the arms or up into the neck. There may be a tingling sensation in the fingers. The patient often clutches his or her chest (Fig. 30). The skin will be grey and perspiring and he or she will appear shocked. There will be dyspnoea and he or she may vomit. The pain will be continuous—unrelieved either by rest or by glycerine trinitrate. The pulse will probably be thin and rapid.

TREATMENT

Arrangements should be made for immediate transport of the patient to hospital. Meanwhile the first-aider should ensure that he or she rests as comfortably as possible—usually this is the semirecumbent position. The pulse and respirations should be checked every 10 to 15 minutes. The patient should not be left unattended and the first-aider should offer calm reassurance. Sips of water may be given if the patient wishes, but alcohol should not be administered.

### Complications of myocardial infarction

Cardiac arrest, cardiogenic shock, cardiac arrhythmias and heart failure are all possible complications of myocardial infarction.

## Cardiogenic shock

Cardiogenic shock is usually the result of a failure in ventricular ejection (often due to massive myocardial infarction) or in ventricular

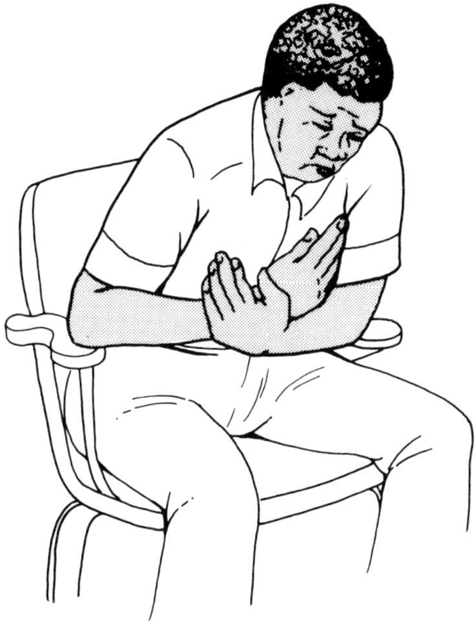

**Fig. 30** Myocardial infarction showing the patient clutching his chest.

filling (as in tamponade) which causes an extremely low cardiac output. The mortality rate is high—85 per cent.

### SIGNS AND SYMPTOMS

The patient is in a severe state of shock and usually unconscious. There is complete peripheral shut down and the peripheries will be cyanosed and cold. The trunk will be cool. Cardiac arrest frequently occurs.

### TREATMENT

The patient must be transferred with the utmost urgency to a hospital and, if available, to an intensive care unit. Meanwhile the first-aider should monitor the patient's heart rate, respirations, skin colour and temperature every 5 minutes. If cardiac arrest occurs, external cardiac massage and artificial respiration must be started at once.

## DISORDERS OF THE CONDUCTING SYSTEM OF THE HEART

The efficient working of the cardiac conducting system is essential for the body to vary its activity. Malfunctions of the system may be confined to the conducting system itself or be manifestations of other cardiac disorders (for example, myocardial infarction).

### Palpitations

Palpitations are the result of tachycardia. Everyone suffers a form of palpitations after violent exercise. If, however, their appearance is unrelated to exercise, there may be some cardiac malfunction (for example, mitral valve disease).

SIGNS AND SYMPTOMS

The patient with palpitations complains of feeling 'the heart pounding in the chest' and will probably appear breathless. The pulse is likely to be irregular, the skin pale and all peripheries cool to touch.

TREATMENT

The first-aider should arrange for the patient to rest—preferably in the semirecumbent position (Fig. 31). If possible she or he should check the apex beat to ascertain the heart rate (in some tachycardias such as atrial fibrillation, many of the beats do not reach the peripheral pulses) and also note the respiratory rate. If the patient has suffered similar attacks previously and recovered quickly, no further action is necessary. If it is the patient's first attack or is a prolonged attack a doctor should be summoned or the patient taken to hospital.

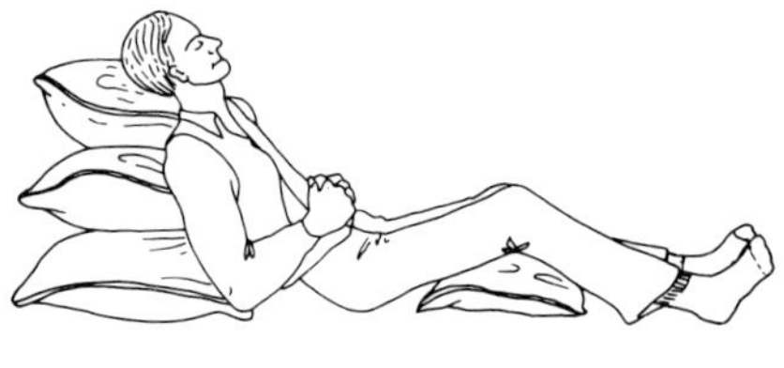

**Fig. 31** The semi-recumbent position. **Note:** Folded coat or cushion under knees to keep patient in position in emergency situation *only*. It should be removed as soon as possible.

### Syncope attacks (Stoke Adams attacks)

Syncope attacks occur as a result of complete heart block in which the conducting mechanism of the heart has failed and few or none of the impulses from the sino-atrial node are reaching the ventricles.

SIGNS AND SYMPTOMS

The patient may complain of feeling tired and breathless, and may have suffered from dizzy spells in the past. He or she may have had no warning of the attack and lose consciousness suddenly. A syncope attack is the result of a short period of asystole due to heart block. Usually the patient recovers spontaneously. If cardiac arrest follows, it should be treated as previously described.

TREATMENT

The first-aider should check the patient's carotid pulse. If the patient's heart is beating and respirations are present, he or she should be placed in the recovery position (Fig. 32) until consciousness is recovered (usually after only a few minutes). Arrangements should be made for immediate transfer to hospital. Meanwhile the pulse and respiration rates should be taken every 15 minutes. The patient is likely to have bradycardia with a pulse rate as low as 20. There are cases, however, where tachycardia and bradycardia may alternate (sick sinus syndrome).

The patient suffering from heart block may also have signs and symptoms of heart failure resulting from cardiac malfunction.

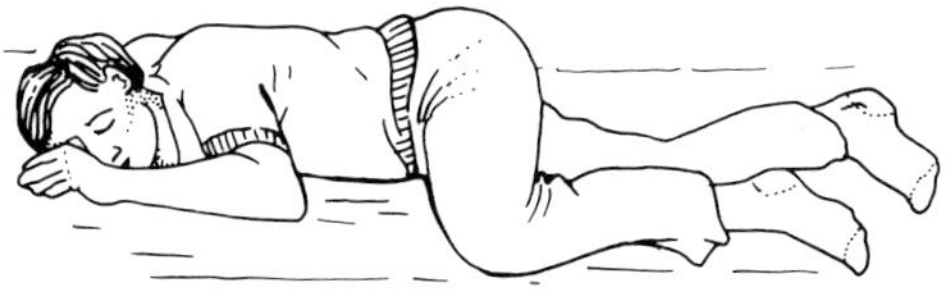

**Fig. 32** The recovery position.

## INJURIES TO THE HEART

Fortunately injuries to the heart are relatively rare. However, with the current increase in violence and road traffic accidents, the first-aider may well have to deal with them.

### Stab wounds and bullet wounds

Stab and bullet wounds may puncture the heart or the great vessels in the mediastinum. If haemorrhage is severe, there is little the first-aider can do to prevent death.

TREATMENT

If the patient who has been stabbed is alive the first-aider should make no attempt to remove the stabbing instrument as it may be acting as a plug and preventing severe haemorrhage. A firm dressing should be placed around the site of entry of the instrument and made as airtight as possible. The first-aider should arrange for immediate transfer of the patient to hospital. If conscious, the patient should be told to lie as still as possible. The heart and respiration rates as well as skin colour should be recorded every 5 minutes. Nothing should be given by mouth.

## Contusion and pericardial effusion

Haemorrhage into the pericardium due to contusion often results from steering wheel injuries and is a complication of flail chest (see page 37). Haemorrhage into the pericardium may lead to tamponade in which the heart becomes so constricted that it is unable to pump properly. The patient will complain of chest pain and appear very shocked. The heart rate will rise whilst the volume of pulses decreases. The patient may lose consciousness, and cardiac arrest may follow.

TREATMENT

The patient should be transferred to hospital immediately. In the meantime the pulse, respirations and skin colour should be observed every 5 to 10 minutes. He or she should be given nothing to eat or drink. Emergency resuscitation procedures should be carried out as necessary.

Pericardial effusion with similar signs and symptoms may also occur after myocardial infarction and should be treated in the same way.

## Aortic aneurysm

Aortic aneurysm may occur following a road traffic accident. It is often associated with steering wheel chest injuries and may occur in cases where there are few obvious serious injuries. The aneurysm is caused by the sudden deceleration which causes the heart to act as a pendulum swinging on the end of the aorta and causing tearing of the aortic wall. The patient complains of considerable central chest pain. He or she may lose consciousness if the aneurysm is a rapidly dissecting one which causes the constriction of the arteries to the brain. If the coronary arteries are affected and the myocardium becomes ischaemic there is little the first-aider can do to prevent cardiac arrest.

TREATMENT

Immediate transfer to hospital should be arranged. The first-aider should observe the patient's pulse, respirations and skin colour as well as the level of consciousness every 5 minutes. If necessary, resuscitation procedures should be carried out. Any other injuries should be dealt with in order of priority.

Because patients may show no outward signs of aortic aneurysm it is advisable that all patients involved in high speed road traffic accidents be sent to hospital for medical examination. If the aneurysm bursts the weakened aortic wall there is little the first-aider can do.

## CARDIAC FAILURE

Cardiac failure exists when the output of the heart is insufficient for the needs of the body. It may be acute or chronic depending on the nature of the underlying causative disease. Cardiac failure due to myocardial infarction will be of more rapid onset than that due to long-standing heart valve disease. The first-aider will be primarily giving aid to cases of acute cardiac failure although she or he may, of course, attend patients suffering from chronic cadiac failure for other reasons. The signs and symptoms of cardiac failure depend on which side of the heart is affected. Left- and right-sided failure frequently coexist.

### Left-sided cardiac failure

When the left side of the heart fails, it is unable to handle blood returning from the lungs and pulmonary oedema therefore develops.

SIGNS AND SYMPTOMS

The patient suffering left-sided cardiac failure will tire easily and

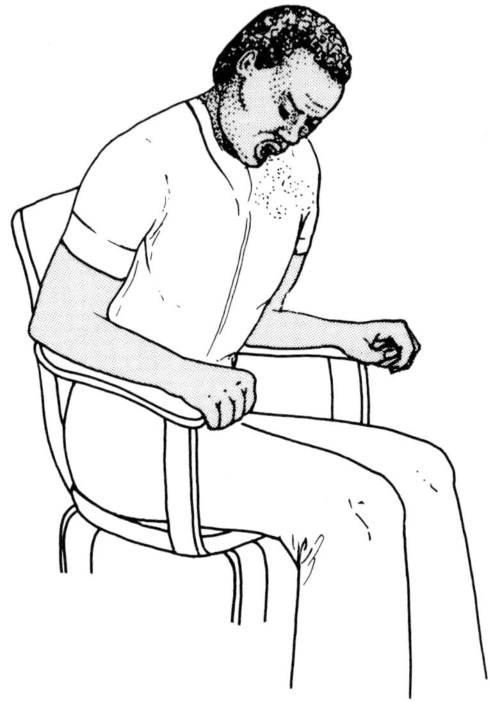

**Fig. 33** Breathlessness in cardiac failure.

appear very breathless (Fig. 33). Copious amounts of watery, frothy sputum may be expectorated. Because of poor exchange of gases in the lungs due to oedema the patient will also be cyanosed. He or she may have chest pain due to either angina or myocardial infarction.

Orthopnoea will cause the patient to become extremely short of breath when lying flat. Patients with cardiac failure often wake up in the night gasping for breath having slipped down off their pillows. (This is also known as cardiac asthma.) They are often extremely anxious and frightened.

TREATMENT

The first-aider should first reassure the patient. If indoors, and the patient is breathless, opening a window will help to give more air. The patient should rest in the semirecumbent position, well supported by pillows. The first-aider should check the pulse and respirations every 30 minutes. If dyspnoea is severe and cyanosis is a feature, the patient should be immediately transferred to hospital. In less severe cases a doctor should be called.

### Right-sided cardiac failure

When the right side of the heart fails, it is unable to cope with blood returning from the systemic circulation. This leads to systemic venous congestion and oedema. Right-sided cardiac failure may occur on its own, but very often it occurs secondary to left-sided cardiac failure.

#### SIGNS AND SYMPTOMS

The patient suffering right-sided cardiac failure therefore exhibits signs of left-sided failure in addition to oedema of the ankles, legs and sacral areas. If the first-aider presses gently on the oedematous area, it will dent and the mark will remain there for a minute or more. This feature is known as 'pitting'.

#### TREATMENT

If there is only systemic oedema and no symptom of pulmonary oedema, the first-aider should arrange for the patient's general practitioner to visit. The patient should be advised to rest and sit with the legs raised. If there is pulmonary oedema, the patient should be treated as for left-sided heart failure.

## DISORDERS OF BLOOD PRESSURE

### Hypertension

The onset of hypertension is usually gradual but the first-aider may become involved in treating some of its more severe manifestations.

#### SIGNS AND SYMPTOMS

The patient may complain of severe headaches and suffer from dizzy spells. He or she will often appear anxious and irritable. Insomnia and fatigue are also features. It is a difficult diagnosis to make without the aid of the sphygmomanometer.

TREATMENT

The patient should lie down in a quiet room. The first-aider should check the pulse and respirations. Tight clothing should be loosened and the patient reassured. A non-alcoholic drink may be given. The patient should be advised to see a doctor as soon as possible.

## Hypotension

Hypotension results from a low cardiac output which is often the result of heart block or cardiac failure. Some people suffer from postural hypotension when they stand up suddenly after lying or bending down; it may also result from standing for a long period without a change of position, for example, soldiers on parade. There is usually no underlying cardiac cause in these cases, but hypotension results from the sudden pull of gravity on the blood, reducing its supply to the brain and upper body.

TREATMENT

The first-aider should lie the dizzy or fainting patient down with the legs raised (Fig. 34). This promotes the supply of blood to vital organs. The pulse and respiration rates should be observed as a low pulse rate may indicate heart block. Tight clothing should be loosened. When the patient has recovered, a drink of water may be given.

If the patient has a bradycardia he or she should be taken to hospital. If suffering from postural hypotension he or she should be helped up

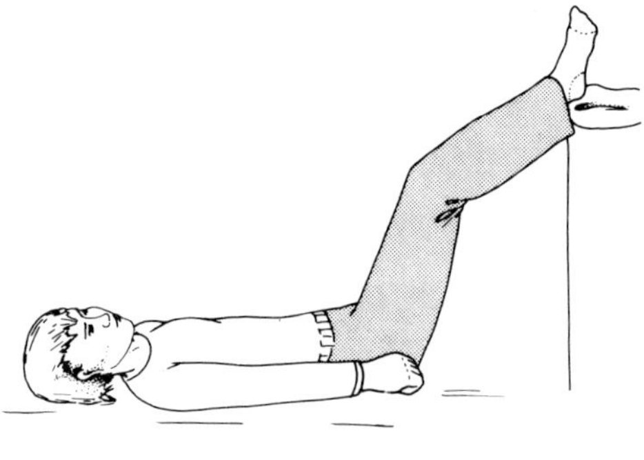

**Fig. 34** Treatment for a dizzy or fainting patient.

slowly from the lying position and advised to visit a general practitioner for a check up as soon as possible.

## VASOVAGAL ATTACKS

Vasovagal attacks are fainting attacks resulting from anxiety, emotional shock (such as being told of the death of a relative), pain or fear. The treatment is as for hypotension and treatment of the underlying cause as necessary, for example, calm reassurance for the anxious person and fresh air when there is a lack of oxygen.

CHAPTER 4

# Trauma I: Shock, Haemorrhage, Wounds and Burns

## SHOCK

Shock is a condition which is the result of insufficient cardiac output with subsequent reduction in the delivery of oxygen to the body cells. It is a life-threatening state requiring immediate recognition and treatment.

The volume of blood varies with age (Fig. 35). Cardiac output is equal to the heart rate multiplied by the volume ejected and this is

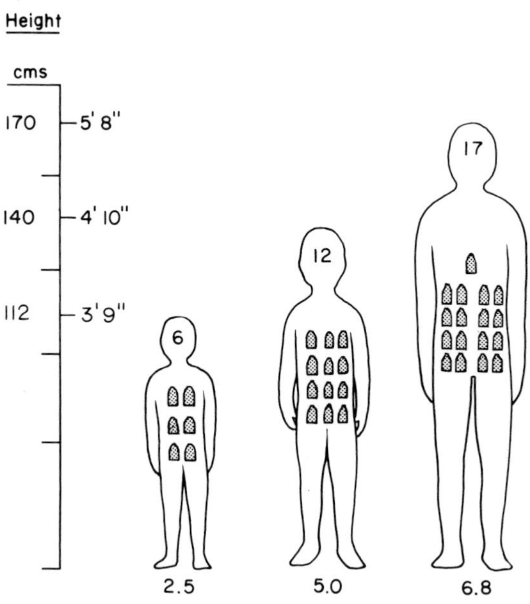


**Fig. 35** The blood volume (in litres) at ages 6, 12 and 17 and the numbers of bottles of blood needed to replace total blood volume.

dependent on a closed system in which the elastic recoil of the aorta, other arteries and arterioles provide the resistance. The blood pressure is thus maintained.

A reduction in cardiac output can therefore be caused by:

- failure of the heart as a pump *or*
- reduction of the circulating volume *or*
- reduced peripheral resistance resulting in a lowered blood pressure

### Failure of the heart to pump

*Cardiogenic* shock occurs following myocardial infarction, particularly when the wall of the left ventricle has been damaged. The heart is unable to pump hard enough to maintain an adequate volume or beat or both. Irregularities of beat or arrhythmias may also occur, causing a futher reduction in heart rate and thus in cardiac output. Fluid or blood in the pericardial sac prevents the heart from filling properly before contraction and effectively reduces the ejection volume (tamponade). (See pages 48–9.)

### Reduction of the circulating blood volume

*Hypovolaemic* shock may occur with loss of whole blood or of plasma. Haemorrhage may be the result of trauma such as the laceration of major vessels and may or may not be obvious straight away. It can also result from disease such as ulcers of the gastrointestinal tract or from a clotting defect in the blood itself.

Severe diarrhoea and vomiting can also cause a rapid reduction of circulating volume, as not only is fluid, which is normally absorbed lost, but fluid intake also ceases.

Plasma loss most commonly occurs following burns or crush injuries. The released cellular metabolites increase the permeability of the capillaries and fluid seeps into the surrounding tissues decreasing the circulating volume.

### Reduced peripheral resistance and reduced blood pressure

When peripheral resistance is lost, vessels dilate allowing pooling of the blood in the capillary bed, a reduction in venous return and, also, eventually, in cardiac output. Severe infections can produce this loss in vascular tone as the circulating toxic substances prevent the nerve endings in the vessel walls responding to impulses from the brain. The vasomotor centre itself may also be affected by these substances.

Fainting is the result of sudden loss of vascular tone, a fall in blood pressure and a subsequent loss of consciousness. As the victim falls to the ground, venous return increases, the blood supply to the brain improves and the vasomotor centre once more becomes active, restoring vasoconstriction and with it an adequate blood pressure.

**Recognition of shock**

The quantity of blood or plasma loss necessary to cause hypovolaemic shock varies between 10 per cent and 20 per cent. The individual's response is related to the time span of the fluid loss, age and general condition of the victim before injury.

Injuries most frequently associated with shock are those leading to blood loss. When loss is obvious—such as bleeding from a limb—the first-aider should try to estimate the amount. Two cupfuls are approximately 10 per cent of the total circulating volume. When internal haemorrhage is suspected, for example, from a chest or abdominal injury, close observation of the patient is necessary for signs and symptoms of shock,

Blunt trauma often leads to serious injuries which result in shock. Blunt trauma to the abdomen—a type of injury which is becoming more common with the increasing use of seat belts—may cause tearing of blood vessels or damage to organs with corresponding loss of blood or plasma. A patient who has this kind of injury in addition to another (such as fractured femur) is very likely to develop hypovolaemic shock.

Other injuries which frequently lead to shock are burns and crush injuries. In both cases, fluid is very rapidly lost into the tissues. In addition, the sudden onset of severe unrelenting pain may disrupt the normal balance between vessel constriction and dilatation. This leads to a fall in blood pressure.

Occasionally traumatic cardiac failure is seen. The most frequent causes of this are blows to the chest, such as those caused by the impact of a steering wheel or a penetrating injury to the chest from a knife or bullet.

SIGNS AND SYMPTOMS

The body has its own mechanism for compensating for a failing circulation, regardless of the cause. It is this mechanism which the first-aider will observe. In an effort to maintain blood pressure to provide perfusion of important organs, such as the brain, heart and lungs, arteriole constriction occurs, initially in the skin, the muscles and the gastrointestinal tract. As this constriction takes place, the patient becomes pale and cold. The skin becomes moist and clammy and perspiration appears on the forehead. (The latter is because sweat glands are stimulated by the same nerves that stimulate blood vessels of the skin.) He or she may also complain of muscle weakness, a dry mouth and thirst.

The pulse rate will increase and become less forceful and respirations will become more rapid. As the delivery of oxygen falls, the patient may become anxious and agitated, but if shock is allowed to progress he or she will become increasingly apathetic.

If the patient remains lying flat, the blood pressure may be maintained. If, however, he or she sits up at this stage, there could be a substantial drop in pressure of 10 per cent or more.

TREATMENT

Arrangements for the patient to be transferred to hospital should be made as soon as possible.

In the meantime, the aim should be to reduce stress from the injury and to prevent the degree of shock from increasing.

The patient should lie flat (Fig. 36) with the head and the trunk level. When possible, cover the patient with a blanket to prevent heat loss. The legs may be slightly elevated to aid venous return. The whole body should not be tipped; this could result in a reduction of blood return from the brain with subsequent cerebral oedema. It could also cause the abdominal organs to fall against the diaphragm thereby impeding respiration.

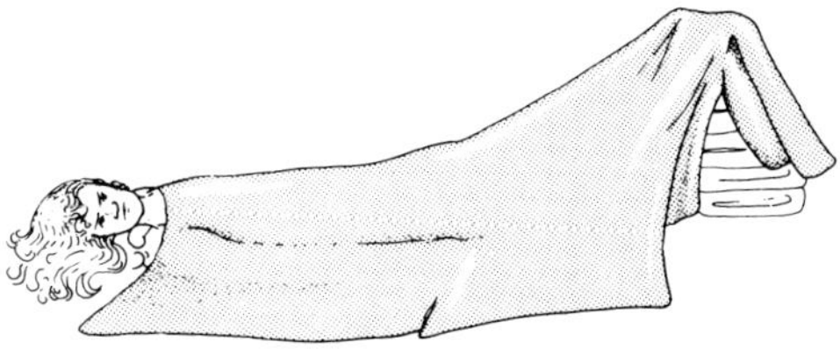

**Fig. 36** Position for the treatment of shock.

If the patient has lost consciousness, the airway must be watched carefully and maintained. If possible he or she should be placed in the recovery position (see Fig. 32, page 51). If this is not possible because of the injuries, the neck should be extended gently to prevent the tongue from falling back (Fig. 37). (See also page 24.)

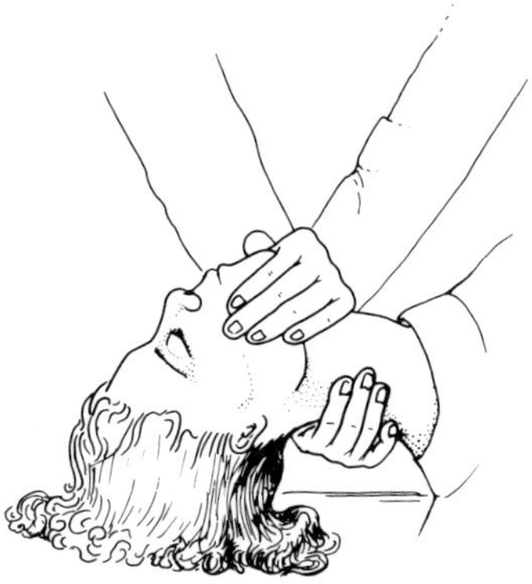

**Fig. 37** Positioning of the head to prevent the tongue blocking the airway.

Haemorrhage should be controlled (see pages 64–8) and fractures immobilised (pages 82–95).

Patients who are shocked often complain of nausea and may vomit. They too, should lie in a position which prevents the possibility of inhaling their vomit.

All movements must be carried out with great care, especially if a brain or spinal injury is suspected (see pages 95–8 and 101–4).

Oxygen may be given if available; it will do no harm and in some instances will prevent further deterioration.

The patient should be protected from additional environmental stresses such as extreme cold or heat. Attempts should be made to allay anxiety.

HOSPITAL MANAGEMENT

Once the patient is in hospital, intravenous fluid replacement will be given and the cause of shock dealt with.

First-aiders must be aware of the possibility of shock developing in all injured people. Quick action in the early stages will prevent the development of profound shock which is sometimes irreversible.

## WOUNDS AND HAEMORRHAGE

A wound is a break in the continuity of the body tissues and may be internal or external.

Wounds are basically destructive injuries and the main objectives in their management are:

- control of bleeding
- treatment of shock
- maintenance of function
- prevention of complications (particularly by reducing the risk of infection)

### Classification of wounds

**Abrasions**

Abrasions are wounds in which the outer layer of skin is scraped away. They are painful and the risk of their becoming infected is high, as foreign material can be ground into the deeper layers of skin and into subcutaneous tissue. Bleeding is usually minimal.

**Punctures**

Punctures are penetrating injuries (Fig. 38a). Causes range from carpet tacks to knives and bullets. Although obvious bleeding is often minimal, internal tissue damage and haemorrhage can be extensive and there is a high infection risk due to the presence of a foreign body.

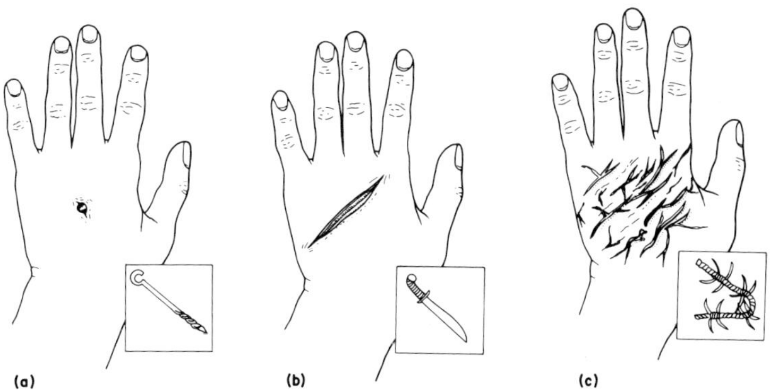


**Fig. 38** Types of wound: (a) punctured, (b) incised and (c) lacerated.

**Avulsions**

Avulsions result when tissues are torn from the body. They are frequently associated with severe bleeding. The scalp may be torn from the skull in a degloving injury (Plate 1). Such a dramatic injury can frequently be repaired with little scarring. If whole parts, for example, ears, fingers, toes, have been torn away they should be taken with the patient to hospital immediately for possible re-attachment.

**Incisions**

Incisions are sharp cuts of variable depth (Fig. 38b). They often bleed severely and there may be damage to underlying structures such as nerves, muscles or tendons. They should be protected against becoming infected as soon as bleeding is controlled.

**Lacerations**

Lacerations are jagged irregular wounds, often involving severe tissue damage (Fig. 38c). They often cause serious bleeding and subsequent hypovolaemic shock.

## Bleeding and its control

Bleeding from a wound can be classified according to the type of vessels damaged.

*Capillary* bleeding results from superficial wounds when blood is said to ooze. Such bleeding is normally controlled by the body's own clotting mechanism. First aid measures may be needed if the wound is extensive. The application of ice compresses can be helpful.

*Venous* bleeding can be recognised when dark red blood flows from a wound. If large veins are involved, this loss may be brisk and life-threatening. Its control should be a priority. Because venous blood is flowing towards the heart, elevating an injured arm or a leg will in the first place, increase the blood flow.

*Arterial* bleeding is bright red in colour and spurts from the wound. It is life-threatening. Its control is secondary to cardiorespiratory arrest only.

There are basically 3 methods for controlling bleeding and they should be used in the following order:

**1** *Direct pressure*
Hard, firm pressure applied directly over the wound is effective in controlling haemorrhage from most wounds (Fig. 39). The pressure should be continued until a firm pressure dressing can be applied.

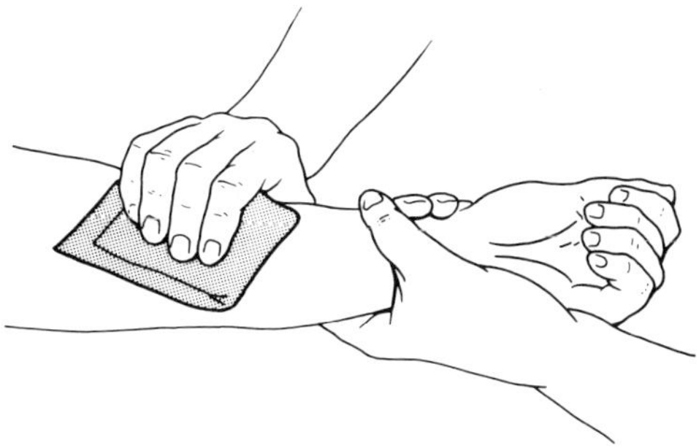

**Fig. 39** Application of direct pressure.

**2** *Arterial pressure*
Should direct pressure not be sufficient to control the bleeding, pressure can be applied to the appropriate arterial pressure point (the point at which the artery is compressed against the underlying bone). Nurses must know the exact location of all these points (Fig. 40).

*Temporal arteries*
The temporal arteries can be located just in front of each ear and may be compressed against the skull to control bleeding from scalp wounds.

*Facial arterial*
Each facial artery can be located just beneath the chin and 2·5 cm in from the angle of the jaw. Pressure applied upwards on to the jaw will control bleeding around the nose and mouth area.

*Common carotid arteries*
The common carotid arteries can be found on either side of the trachea. Pressure here can be applied against muscles but only if no other method is effective. Pressure dressings should never be applied. Extreme care must be taken and pressure applied only for a very short time during which the patient's airway must be carefully watched. Pressure should *never* be applied to both carotid arteries at the same time.

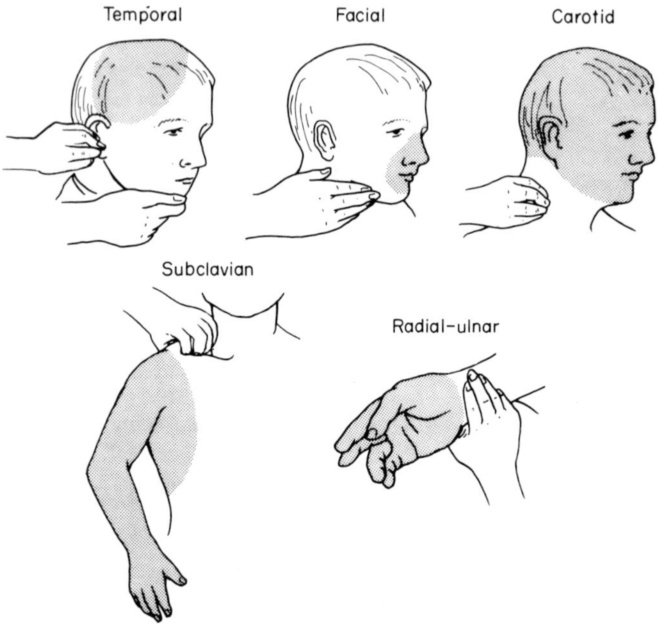


**Fig. 40** Location of arterial pressure points and the areas served.

*Subclavian arteries*

The subclavian arteries are situated just under the clavicle (collar bone) on either side, and supply that area and also the upper shoulders. Pressure should be applied downwards just behind and about half way along the clavicle. When the artery is successfully occluded, the patient will complain of numbness in the arm and hand and the radial pulse will be absent.

*Brachial arteries*

The brachial arteries supply the lower arms and hands and are situated on the inner aspect of the upper arms between the biceps and triceps muscles (Fig. 41). Approximately one-third of the way from the shoulder to the elbow, a pulse may be felt. Pressure should be applied at that point.

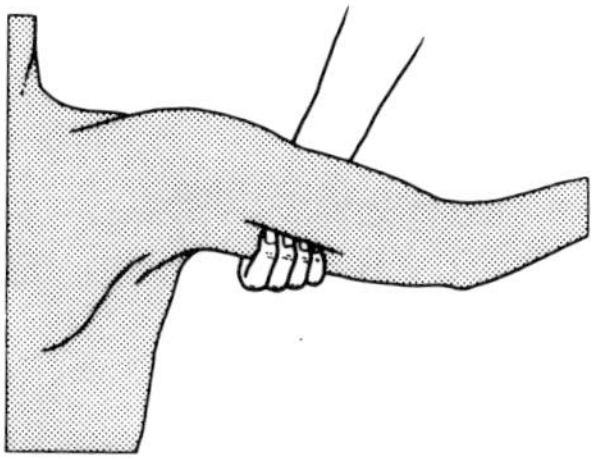

**Fig. 41** Application of pressure to the brachial pulse.

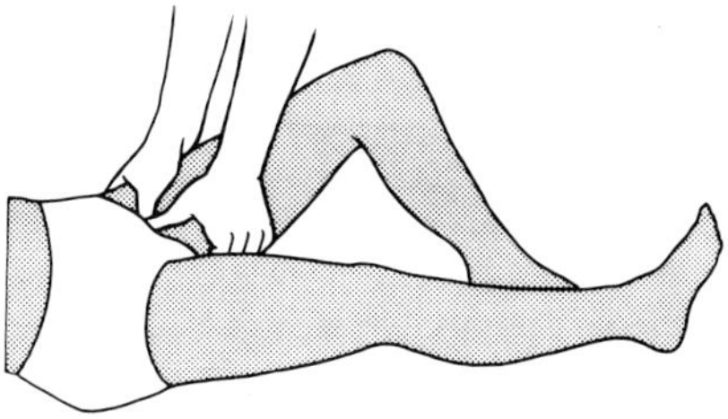

**Fig. 42** Application of pressure to the femoral pulse.

*Femoral arteries*
Pulses from the femoral arteries can be felt in the groins (Fig. 42). Bleeding from these arteries can be very severe, and the first-aider should be able to locate and occlude them rapidly and effectively.

*Radial and ulnar arteries*
The radial artery can be located on the surface of the wrist on the thumb side and the ulnar artery on the opposite anterior side. These should be compressed together to arrest severe bleeding from the hand until a pressure dressing can be firmly applied.

In cases of very severe bleeding, manual pressure over the main artery proximal to the bleeding point should be applied as well as direct pressure over the wound itself whenever possible.

The method is limited, however, by the difficulty of maintaining adequate pressure for any length of time and the difficulty of keeping the pressure applied during movement and transport of the patient. A disadvantage is that it does not control bleeding from collateral vessels. In the event of mass casualties, it is a method which is uneconomical in the use of helpers as it monopolises the attention or expertise of the nurse at the expense of other victims. It is sometimes helpful, however, to instruct a helper to apply pressure on an artery whilst a dressing is being applied to the wound.

**3** *Tourniquets*
The use of a tourniquet is hazardous and bleeding can almost always be controlled by other means. The decision to apply a tourniquet is a

decision to risk a limb in order to save a life. In general there is no place for the use of tourniquets in first aid practice except for treatment of bleeding amputation stumps (very rare indeed).

The first-aider who applies a tourniquet has a moral obligation to stay with the patient in order to release it for 5 minutes every 20 minutes and to see that it is removed after 2 hours.

The main disadvantages of a tourniquet are:

The construction of the tourniquet causes pain which adds to the patient's restlessness.

If applied too tightly, uninjured tissues may be damaged, especially nerves and blood vessels.

If applied too loosely, bleeding is increased as only the venous circulation is shut down and arterial blood pours into the limb from which it cannot return.

It may be applied and forgotten.

*Rules to follow when applying a tourniquet*

**1** Use appropriate material, cloth or stocking or tie, never wire or rope.

**2** Apply just above the site of the wound and tighten sufficiently to stop bleeding.

**3** Note time of application and mark this on the patient.

**4** Do not cover the tourniquet.

**5** Transport the patient to medical care immediately.

**6** Treat for shock in the meantime.

*Application*

The appropriate material should be wrapped twice around the injured limb and tied tightly. A suitable strong object should be placed between the two layers of material close to the knot and turned, tightening the outer layer until the bleeding has stopped. It should then be made secure, using the ends of the material. **Do not cover.**

## Management of wounds

### Minor wounds

Minor wounds involve only the superficial layers of skin. These should be cleaned and may be dressed if necessary, using a commercial dressing impregnated with antiseptic. The first-aider should not forget the importance of washing her or his own hands when dealing with these minor injuries.

Some relatively minor wounds require suturing, and in this case the patient should be taken to a doctor. Until then, the wound should be cleaned and a clean dry dressing applied. Cleansing can often be effectively achieved by putting the wound under a running tap. A freshly laundered handkerchief or tea-towel with the unfolded inside surface placed next to the wound may be used as an improvised dressing.

**Major wounds**

If possible the area around a major wound should be cleaned. If the wound itself has foreign material ground into it, this should be removed only if it can be done simply and without probing. A clean dressing should be applied over the wound and the patient transferred to hospital without delay.

**Abdominal wounds**

An abdominal wound should be treated as described above and the patient monitored for shock until he or she arrives at hospital. Internal bleeding may well occur into the peritoneal cavity with little obvious sign to begin with. Close scrutiny will reveal slight bruising (Plate 2) and this may be the only sign of a serious internal injury.

HOSPITAL MANAGEMENT

Penetrating wounds of the abdomen require exploratory laparotomy to discover the extent of the damage and repair it.

*Evisceration of the abdominal organs*

The first-aider should not try to replace protruding viscera. A sterile dressing saturated with normal saline (if not available, tap water may be used) should be applied and kept moist until medical help is reached. The patient should be placed flat and kept as still as possible. No fluids should be given. Treatment for shock may be required (see pages 58–62).

## Chest injuries

Injuries to the chest are dealt with in Chapter 1.

## Head injuries

First aid procedures for injuries of the head and neck are described in Chapter 5.

## Eye injuries

If a foreign body enters the eye at speed it may perforate the cornea and remain inside the eye. The condition is usually very painful and serious, so immediate admission to hospital is required. Meanwhile, the first-aider should do as little as possible. The patient will probably close his or her injured eye because of the pain.

### TREATMENT

With eye injuries, a *very light* covering, for example, a clean handkerchief, may be applied but great care should be taken not to increase the pressure as this could cause the extrusion of the intraocular contents. On *no account* should the eye be irrigated. Intraocular foreign bodies are often found following a windscreen injury (Plate 3), when pieces of glass enter the eye causing it to swell.

## Bleeding

The causes of bleeding from certain sites of the body may not always be immediately apparent to the first-aider, for example, from the ear and the nose. All bleeding must be attended to promptly whether or not the causes are obvious. A tooth socket, for example, may bleed some time after a tooth has been removed. The following treatments also include bleeding from the tongue or cheek, from varicose veins and from the palm of the hand.

### TREATMENT: BLEEDING FROM THE EAR

Cover the ear with clean (sterile, if available) dressing and apply bandage.

Do **not** plug the ear with wool.
Do **not** instil ear drops.
Refer the patient for investigation.

If the bleeding follows a blow on the head, lay the patient down with the head inclined towards the affected side. Remove the patient to hospital as soon as possible.

### TREATMENT: BLEEDING FROM THE NOSE

Instruct the patient to pinch the lower part of his or her nose firmly for 10 minutes, breathing through the mouth (Fig. 43).

Sit the patient by an open window with his or her head bent slightly forward over a bowl.

Loosen tight clothing around the neck.

Warn the patient not to blow his or her nose for several hours.

If bleeding persists, or recurs, send to the doctor.

### TREATMENT: BLEEDING FROM A TOOTH SOCKET

Sit the patient down.

Put a small pad of lint or gauze over, but not deeply in the socket. This should be large enough to keep upper and lower teeth apart when bitten on.

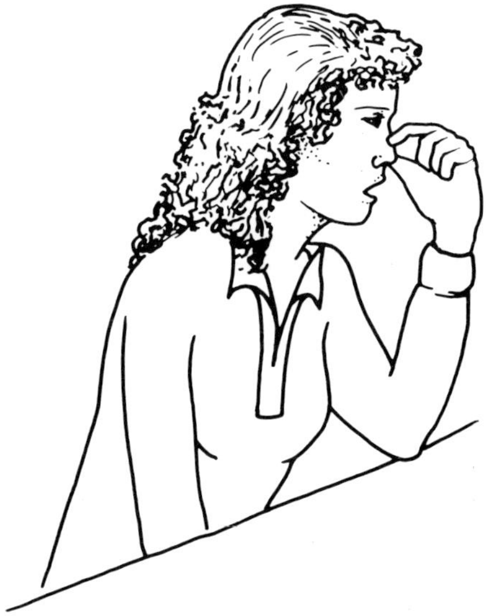

**Fig. 43** Treatment for a nose bleed.

Tell the patient to bite hard on this pad for 15 minutes, supporting the chin with his or her hand.

If bleeding persists, or recurs, send to the dentist.

TREATMENT: BLEEDING FROM THE TONGUE OR CHEEK

Compress the part between the finger and thumb, using a clean handkerchief or dressing, if available.

TREATMENT: BLEEDING FROM VARICOSE VEINS

Immediately press hard with the hand over the bleeding part until a dressing is available.

Lay the patient down with the affected leg raised.

Cover the bleeding part with a dry dressing and pad, and bandage firmly.

Remove any garter or other constriction above the bleeding point.

Prevent shock.

Refer patient to hospital.

TREATMENT: BLEEDING FROM THE PALM OF THE HAND

Apply direct pressure.

Raise the limb.

If no fracture or irremovable foreign body is present the first-aider should then:

Cover the wound with a clean dressing or handkerchief.

Place a pad over the dressing.

Bend the fingers over the pad.

Bandage the fist firmly with a folded triangular bandage tying off across the knuckles.

Support the affected limb in a triangular sling.

**Bandages and bandaging**

A bandage has two main purposes; first, to keep a splint or dressing in place and, second, to apply pressure.

*Retentive bandages*

Any material which can be made to encircle the part to keep a dressing in place can be used: a scarf, stocking or tie, as well as the more usual triangular bandage found in first aid kits.

*Pressure bandages*
Firm, even pressure is best applied by a crêpe bandage that is fairly well stretched as it is being applied. Even distribution of pressure is maintained by applying the bandage over a thick layer of wool extending well over the wound.

Elastic bandages containing rubber require special caution; they should be stretched only slightly when being applied, and if possible, should be avoided altogether.

*Emergency dressings*
Emergency dressings can be made from clean linen or a towel or handkerchief. Hold up the material by its corners and allow it to fall open; then refold it without touching the surface which previously was inside, but which is now on the outside. Secure in place by using any suitable article to hand such as a scarf or stocking.

Shell dressings for large wounds consist of gauze, cotton wool and attached bandage.

**Crush syndrome**
A casualty who has been trapped by wreckage of any kind poses a number of problems; the most important decision to make is whether life is immediately endangered. This could be by fire, explosion, crushing of trunk, or head—or the likelihood that any of these may happen—by loss of blood and by suffocation. Speedy and sometimes forcible extraction is justified but there should not be frantic, thoughtless haste. It is important to distinguish between courage and folly in disaster situations and to recognise the dangers as well as the difficulties.

The crush syndrome results from severe and prolonged crushing of limbs. It is characterised by renal failure following the profound hypotension, which has been caused by great loss of blood into the crushed tissues after they have been released.

Myoglobin and other products of disrupted tissues can be present without detriment to the kidneys providing the blood pressure is restored to normal quickly by liberal blood transfusion.

If the limb has been crushed for 3 to 4 hours or more, or is so badly injured as to be irrecoverable, a tight tourniquet should be applied as near as possible to the proximal edge of the crushed part, preferably before release. This tourniquet can be left in place until the limb is amputated (which may be necessary in order to free the patient). The tourniquet will prevent the loss of liquids into the crushed limb and the escape into the bloodstream of myoglobin and other products of anoxia and injury.

If the limb has been crushed for a short time and if there is a chance of recovery and repair, it should be bandaged firmly (if other injuries permit) in order to try to prevent excessive swelling. A tourniquet should not be used unless there is severe bleeding which cannot be controlled in any other way.

If there is much delay in getting the victim removed to hospital, the conscious patient may be offered water to drink; small quantities at first and larger quantities if well tolerated. Although this will do virtually nothing to raise the blood pressure, it will help to replenish the body's depleted water content. If the crushed limb has been amputated or excluded by a tourniquet or if the patient is within 15 minutes' reach of hospital, there is no need to encourage copious drinking.

**Replacing blood loss**

Unfortunately group O rhesus negative blood, which can be given safely without preliminary grouping and matching, is too scarce to be carried by emergency teams as a matter of course.

Plasma can be given, if available, but usually this is possible only in hospital.

The next most satisfactory intravenous fluid is either dextran (which acts as a plasma expander by increasing the osmotic pressure, and drawing in extracellular fluid), Hartmann's solution or normal saline. However, erecting an intravenous infusion at the site of an accident where first aid is being carried out does carry a high risk of infection.

**Haemostatic agents**

Although a wide range of substances which control bleeding exist, many are not suitable for first aid practice. If available, gelatin sponge, fibrin foam or thrombin topical can be applied to a large area of capillary oozing.

**Assessment of blood loss**

Whilst nurses will be able to recognise exsanguination and the signs and symptoms of severe bleeding, it is important also for them to try to estimate the volume of blood which has been lost at the site of the accident (Fig. 44).

A blood donor gives about 10 per cent of blood volume with little effect. More than 10 per cent loss causes tachycardia. If the patient has tachycardia but a normal blood pressure, the loss will not be more than 20 per cent of the blood volume.

If, however there is also a falling blood pressure and the extremities are pale and cool, then the loss is probably nearer 30 per cent. The patient may appear fairly fit at this stage but even just a slightly increased loss may quickly produce collapse. Such a collapse could be precipitated by injudicious handling, anaesthesia, manipulation of

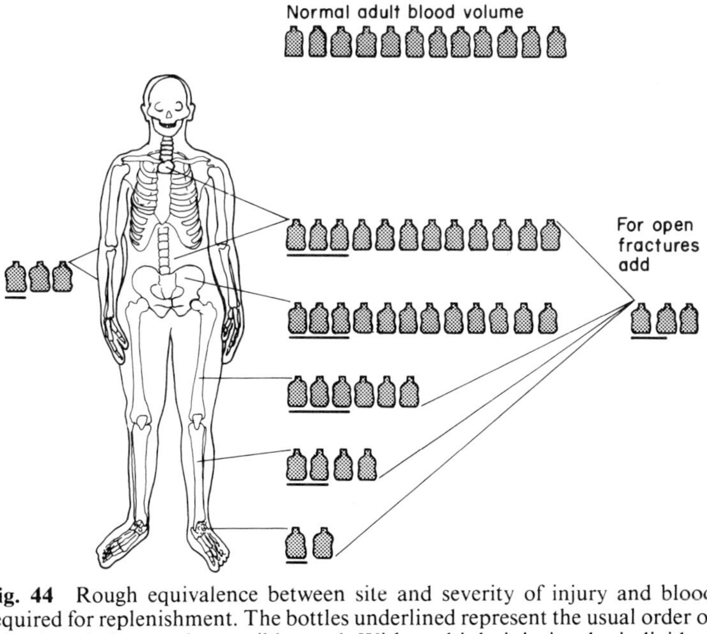


**Fig. 44** Rough equivalence between site and severity of injury and blood required for replenishment. The bottles underlined represent the usual order of loss, the whole row the possible need. With multiple injuries the individual losses have to be added and may considerably exceed a blood volume.

broken bones or a long journey to hospital. This latent shock is an important state to recognise.

The size of a wound in closed injuries is indicated roughly by the size of the swelling, but it is not only the size that is important—the area it occupies is significant also. Bruising also gives an indication of the amount of blood loss (Plate 4).

In the case of an open wound, some attempt should be made to assess the volume of blood lost at the scene of the accident, on the clothes, seats of motor cars, coaches, and so on. In abdominal and pelvic injuries the assessment of oligaemic shock is more difficult. A patient with a severe fracture of the pelvis may lose up to 3 litres of blood fairly quickly and up to 10 litres if transfusion is initiated and bleeding not controlled.

## BURNS

Burns damage the skin and constitute a break in the skin surface. They can therefore be defined as a wound.

The skin is one of the largest organs in the body comprising 16 per cent of the total body weight. Skin provides:

Sensory protection.
Thermo regulation.
Fluid retention.
Protection against bacteria and other organisms.

When skin is burned all these functions are disturbed.

### Classification of burns

#### Thermal burns

Thermal burns can be caused by dry or wet heat. If the latter, they are called scalds.

#### Corrosive chemical burns

Corrosive chemicals, strong acids and alkalis can cause severe and extensive damage. Hydrofluoric acid is widely used in industry and is also added to the water used by window-cleaning contractors to clean roof lights. There are, therefore, many chances of being burned. Concentrated hydrofluoric acid causes skin lesions varying from erythema to severe burns. It infiltrates tissues rapidly and deeply. Systemic fluoride poisoning can occur from extensive burns. Droplets of anhydrous hydrofluoric acid cause penetrating burns in direct proportion to their size. Pain, which may be delayed, is severe. The burned area is red at first and later becomes blanched in the centre. If not treated, it progresses to necrosis.

### Electrical burns

Electrical burns are usually less extensive but deep. Patients sustaining electrical burns may also suffer cardiac arrest due to the passage of thc current through the heart.

The first-aider must ensure that the patient is no longer in contact with the current before touching him or her. If it is not possible to switch the current off, the patient should be removed from it, using clothing or a non-metal implement such as a walking stick. If cardiac arrest has occurred energetic resuscitation should be carried out.

### Irradiation burns

Irradiation burns are rare. Their development is slow and their treatment usually carried out on an out-patient basis.

## The severely burned patient

The severity of the burn depends largely on two factors:

the depth of the burn (Plate 5)
the extent of the burn

### The depth of the burn

Burns are described as superficial, partial thickness or full thickness (or first, second or third degree) (Fig. 45).

*Superficial* burns involve only the outer layer of epithelium and give rise to blisters and erythema (Plate 6). They are painful, due to irritation of the nerve endings. They usually heal within 2 to 3 days and without treatment.

*Partial thickness* burns cause damage to the deeper layer of epidermis thus exposing a red, weeping area of the capillary bed (Plate 7). They form blisters and are painful. If kept clean they too will heal

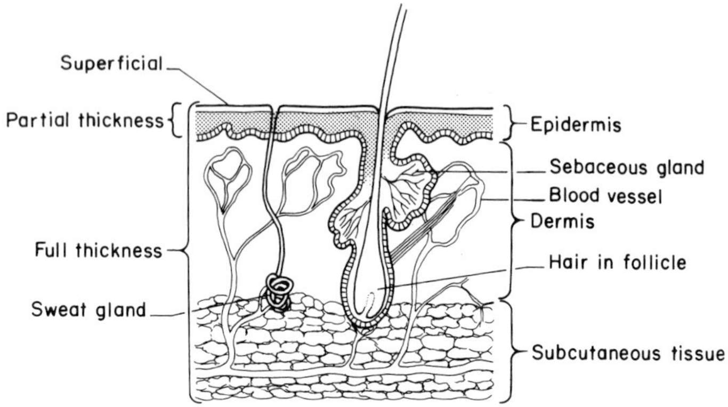


**Fig. 45** The skin and the various depths of burns.

over a period of 1 to 4 weeks without treatment and with little or no scarring. Erythema may remain for a longer time. If a partial thickness burn becomes infected, however, the remaining delicate skin will be destroyed resulting in a full thickness burn.

*Full thickness* burns involve complete destruction of the skin including the germinal layer. The area looks dry, firm and charred and will be painless because nerve endings are destroyed. Very severe full thickness burns can destroy the subcutaneous tissue to reveal the muscle fascia (Plate 8).

Differentiation between partial and full thickness burns is very hard at this stage. But it is as well to remember that if even partial thickness burns become infected, further damage can occur and full thickness skin destroyed thus necessitating skin grafting at a later date.

**The extent of the burn**

The extent of the burn is classically calculated by using the rule of 9, which divides the body into areas approximately 9 per cent of its whole (Fig. 46).

Any burn greater than 15 per cent in adults or 10 per cent in children, should be transferred to hospital immediately. Patients with burns affecting smaller areas of the hands, feet, face and genitalia should also be transferred to hospital.

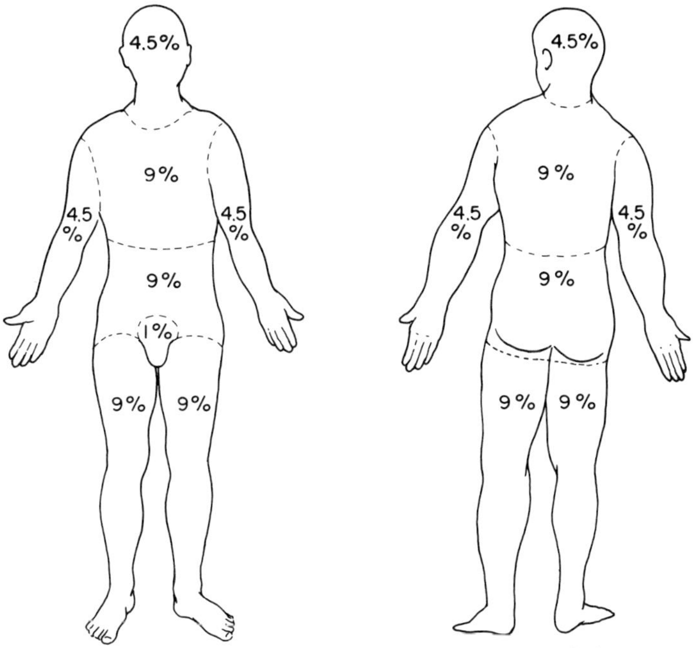


**Fig. 46** The rule of nine used to calculate the extent of a burn.

TREATMENT

If clothes are on fire:

Put out the flames with cold water if this is to hand.

If water is not available, smother the flames by laying the patient down and wrapping a blanket, coat or rug very tightly round him or her.

Tear off smouldering clothes by seizing non-affected areas of the material.

If available at the scene at the time of burning or scalding, immerse or flood the burned part in cold water.

Remove any clothing soaked in boiling water. **Do not** remove burned clothing which has cooled.

Remove any constrictions such as rings, bracelets or boots before the affected part begins to swell.

Cover lightly with a sterile or clean cloth or sheet.

**Do not**

handle the burned area
prick any blisters
apply lotion or ointment
remove debris

If the burns are severe, remove the patient to hospital immediately.

**Corrosive chemicals**

Flood the area at once with copious running water, protecting unaffected parts.

Remove contaminated clothing, avoiding contamination of yourself.

Treat affected area as a wound.

**Extensive burns**

An extensively burned patient should be wrapped in a clean sheet; kept warm with blankets, if necessary; and taken immediately to hospital.

The supreme need is early adequate transfusion; local treatment takes second place. The loss of fluid from the system into the surrounding tissues is due to increased capillary permeability and will lead to shock and gross oedema (Plate 9). Severe oedema may cause respiratory difficulty by direct tightness over the chest as well as swelling of the throat. The surgeon may split the skin to release the pressure.

It will enable hospital staff to calculate the amount and rate of replacement fluid if the first-aider is able to tell them:

the time the patient was burned
the cause of the burn
the percentage of the burn

Any associated injury should also be noted, especially if the casualty has been removed from an enclosed, smoke-filled space. Respirations should be closely observed for signs of obstruction which can occur from inhalation of smoke and debris or damage (by heat) of the upper respiratory tract. In extreme cases a tracheostomy may need to be performed.

**Minor burns and scalds**

Minor burns and scalds can usually be treated effectively by placing the affected area under running cold water.

If a tap is not available, immersion in ice-cold water will help to alleviate heat and pain. The casualty should be instructed to repeat this procedure at 3 to 4 minute intervals until the burn is no longer painful out of water.

## COLD INJURY

Just as extreme heat can damage the tissues of the body so can extreme heat loss, or cold (see Plates 15–17). Cold injury can be classified as to whether all or only a part of the body is involved.

Frostbite is the destruction of the tissues by freezing, and occurs most commonly on the nose, cheeks, ears, fingers and toes. The surrounding area is also damaged. The frozen area becomes black and is usually small, but before this stage is reached, the area may redden and the skin then turns greyish or white. At this point it may be painful but later this subsides. People may be unaware that they have frostbite until it is brought to their attention by others who notice the grey or white patch that appears on the cheek, for example.

Treatment begins by preventing further heat loss with the use of dry clothing as insulating garments and by seeking shelter. Drugs which affect the peripheral vascular system or impair judgement or both should be avoided.

Apply extra protection in the form of dry clothes or blankets while transporting the patient to a protected environment where he or she can be given a warm drink if conscious. Rewarm the frozen part rapidly by placing it in warm water (38·9–40·6° C if thermometer available) until it becomes flushed. With slow thawing, tissue damage increases. The patient should be encouraged to exercise the area although massage should not be applied. Medical aid should be sought as soon as possible. In the meantime, dressings may be applied after the area has been gently cleansed in warm soapy water. Blisters should not be broken nor should additional heat be applied. Jewellery should be removed in anticipation of swelling.

While cold injury is considered trauma, it is the result of exposure; other aspects of frostbite and its treatment are described on pages 157–8.

## CHAPTER 5

# Trauma II: Musculoskeletal Injuries

There are ten general principles to be observed in the management of major trauma:

**1** Treat the patient on the spot unless it is dangerous to do so.
**2** Maintain a clear airway.
**3** Control bleeding.
**4** Be aware that while carrying out emergency care, further injury can be caused. (This is particularly relevant when caring for patients with injuries to the central nervous system. Mismanagement can lead to death or disability.)
**5** Support and reassure the injured patient.
**6** Cover any open wound.
**7** Do not try to push back protruding bone.
**8** Immobilise fractured limbs.
**9** Continue to monitor the patient's condition from the time of injury until the time he or she reaches hospital.
**10** Keep the patient as comfortable as possible.

Injuries to the musculoskeletal system are generally not life-threatening but many relatively minor injuries are potentially dangerous. Informed care by the nurse can prevent serious complications resulting in permanent damage and disability.

## FRACTURES

A fracture is a break in the continuity of bone and is usually the result of violence in one form or another. Those caused by direct violence are fractures in which the break occurs at the point of impact. Indirect violence is said to be the cause when the fracture occurs some distance from the blow; for example, when a fractured ulnar or radius is the result of a fall on to the outstretched hand. Stress fractures occur in athletes sometimes and heal spontaneously with rest. Pathological fractures occur when the bone is already weakened by disease: even a very small amount of stress can cause it to break.

## Classification

Fractures in which there is no break in the skin are described as closed or simple (Fig. 47a); when the skin is broken they are open or compound. The skin break can be as a result of damage by something external, occurring simultaneously with a fracture, or it can be caused by the end of a broken bone perforating the skin (Fig. 47b).

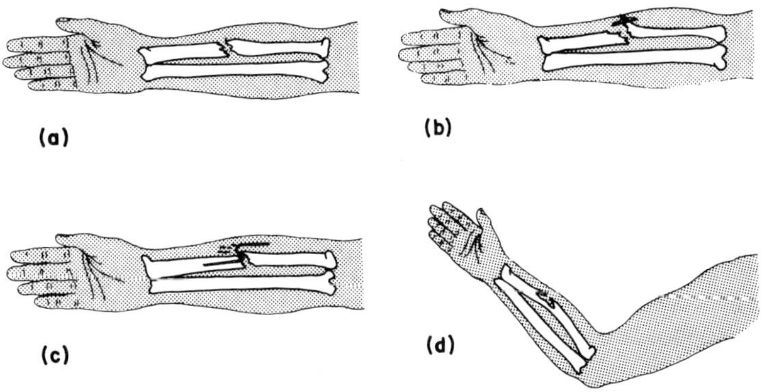


**Fig. 47** Types of fracture: (a) closed, (b) open, (c) complicated and (d) greenstick.

A fracture may also be complicated. This is when there is damage to other tissues (Fig. 47c). This possibility should be taken into account when treating a patient with fractured ribs (possible lung damage) or a skull fracture (possible brain damage). The first-aider must also remember that relatively straightforward fractures of the limbs may be complicated by damage to major blood vessels and nerves. A greenstick fracture can occur in childhood when the bone is only partly broken (Fig. 47d).

SIGNS AND SYMPTOMS

Signs and symptoms will vary according to the site of injury. If there is any doubt as to whether or not the patient has a fracture the first-aider should assume that he or she has and treat accordingly. This rule is particularly relevant when there is severe swelling.

The casualty should be asked if he or she has any pain. If so, the first-aider should then examine the painful area for swelling and deformity. It is helpful to compare both sides of the body when doing this. Abnormal angles and positions or limb shortening should also be looked for. Crepitus or grating can be heard when bone ends rub against each other, but this should not be deliberately looked for. The patient should always be asked to keep as still as possible to prevent increasing the injury.

A certain amount of bleeding into the tissues around a fracture is inevitable and sometimes this is considerable. When it happens, the patient should be placed flat in order to prevent shock developing from blood loss and pain.

#### TREATMENT

The patient should be treated where he or she is, unless the patient and the first-aider are in danger. There should be as little movement as possible. If the fracture is open and there is severe bleeding this should be dealt with first, and a dressing applied. Direct pressure is usually sufficient although the patient may not be able to tolerate this, in which case the appropriate arterial pressure point may need to be used. The wound should be covered by a sterile dressing.

The fracture should then be immobilised. This can be done by immobilising the joint above and below the fracture. The first-aider must ensure that when any types of splint are used, they must be padded where they come into contact with the body and that they do not interfere with normal circulation. The patient should then be placed on a stretcher and transported to hospital. Elevating the fractured limb during the journey not only aids the prevention of shock, but also reduces swelling of the injured part.

### Use of bandages

Bandages must be applied sufficiently firmly to prevent movement but not so tightly as to interfere with the circulation or cause pain.

In order to prevent chafing and discomfort of the skin, skin surfaces should be separated with soft padding before bandaging.

Always tie knots over a splint or on the uninjured side. If both lower limbs are injured, tie the knots in front and between them.

Check at 15 minute intervals to ensure that bandages are not becoming too tight as the result of swelling of injured tissues. (This is especially important when an injured elbow is supported in a sling.)

When it is necessary to pass bandages under the casualty do so by using the natural hollows of the body—neck, knees and ankles.

## Use of splints

The first-aider should be content with rendering the limb comfortable and steady enough to allow the casualty to be transported without undue disturbance and pain. This is all that is required to stay the progress of shock. Formal splintage is not necessarily the best way of achieving this objective. Inflatable splints offer a valuable combination of simplicity, comfort and efficacy. Only for long, rough journeys is elaborate splinting justified. Well-judged restraint is preferable to lavishing treatment on any and every injury.

Inflatable splints should be used if available. All splints should be:

- sufficiently rigid
- long enough to immobilise the joint both above and below the fracture
- well-padded (if not inflatable), and wide enough to fit the limb comfortably
- applied over clothing

In emergencies, splints may be improvised by using walking sticks, umbrellas, broom handles, pieces of wood, cardboard, rolled newspaper or thick, firmly folded bandages. The patient's body can also be used as a splint sometimes and with a combination of improvisations a satisfactory immobilisation can usually be achieved.

## The skull

SIGNS AND SYMPTOMS

There may be blood loss from the ear or nose. Sometimes this is swallowed and later vomited.

TREATMENT

Initiate resuscitation procedures, if necessary.

Place the casualty in the recovery position.
Establish the level of consciousness.
Apply and secure a sterile dressing over the ear if there is a loss of fluid from it.
Remove the patient quickly and carefully to hospital.

When a fractured skull is suspected, the casualty should be kept quiet and his head slightly elevated. If any abnormal depression of the skull is seen pressure should not be applied as this could cause brain damage. More detailed care of a patient with a fractured skull or head injury or both can be found on pages 101–4.

## The jaw

SIGNS AND SYMPTOMS

Usually only one side of the jaw is broken. There may be pain, which is increased by jaw movements or swallowing; excessive flow of saliva which is often blood-stained; irregularity of teeth; swelling and tenderness of the lower face; and, if the tongue is involved, haemorrhage from the mouth.

TREATMENT

Maintain an airway, removing any detached or false teeth.
Control bleeding.
Support the jaw with a soft pad and suitable bandage (Fig. 48).
If unconscious, place the casualty in the recovery position on the uninjured side, keeping the jaw well forward.
Remove to hospital as soon as possible.

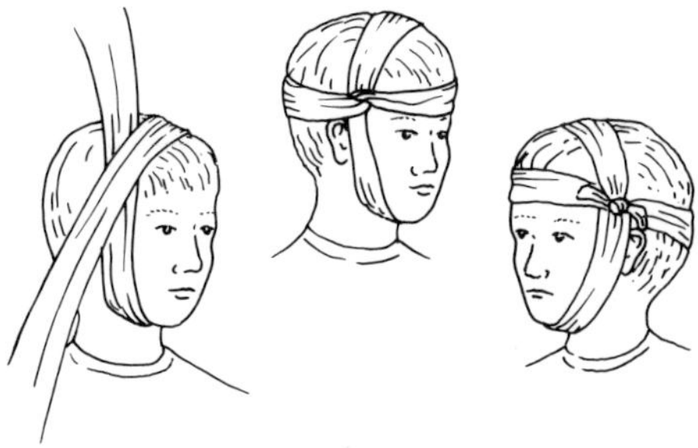

**Fig. 48** The bandaging of a fractured jaw, firmly supportive but not tightly constricting. This should only be used on a fully conscious casualty when there is no likelihood of vomiting.

## The sternum

Fracture of the sternum is usually associated with crush injuries and may be complicated by damage to underlying organs.

TREATMENT
Loosen any tight clothing around neck, chest and waist. Place casualty in semirecumbent position if this is fairly comfortable. Transport by stretcher to hospital.

## The clavicle

A fractured clavicle is usually caused by falling on to an outstretched hand. Only occasionally will it be the result of a direct blow. The casualty will probably present with the injured arm supported by the other hand. The casualty's head may be inclined towards the injured side, thereby relieving the pain by reducing muscle tension. There may be swelling or deformity at the site of the fracture.

TREATMENT
Narrowly fold 2 triangular bandages.

Pass each under one axilla, encircle the shoulder and tie behind in a reef knot.

Carry the free ends of the bandages across the casualty's back and over a pad placed between the shoulder blades.

Tie opposite ends or secure with a third bandage. Support the arm on the injured side in another triangular sling.

In practice, a deformity is usually accepted and some surgeons go so far as to dispense with any form of support, encouraging active use for the whole limb right from the start. It is sufficient, therefore, to promote comfort by bracing the shoulders back and placing the arm in a sling.

## The humerus

A fractured humerus or upper arm is best immobilised by using the upper part of the body as a splint. If the elbow is not involved, the arm should be gently bent at the elbow and a sling applied (Fig. 49a). It should then be secured to the body, using bandages, scarves, ties and

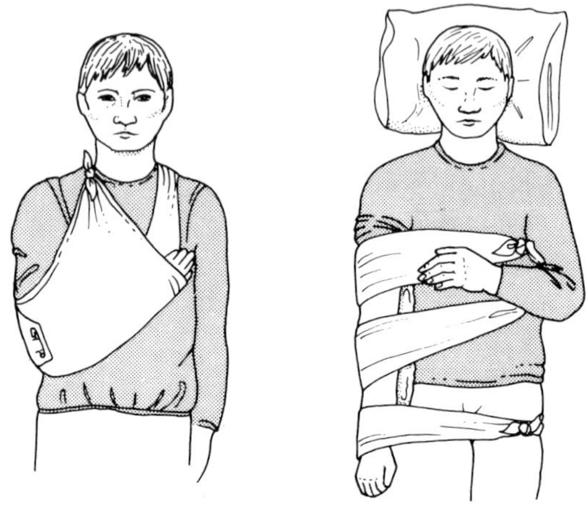

(a) (b)

**Fig. 49** Treatment of a fractured humerus when (a) the elbow is not involved and (b) in a reclining position when the elbow cannot be flexed.

the like; one placed below the fracture and one above. It is worth noting that if nothing suitable is available for making a sling, the patient's clothing can be used by pinning the sleeve to the front of the jacket on the opposite side.

If the elbow cannot be flexed (Fig. 49b):

Do not force flexion of the elbow.

Lay the casualty down.

Gently position the arm by the casualty's side, palm to thigh.

Place adequate soft padding between the arm and body.

Secure with 3 broad bandages tied on the uninjured side of the body:

round the upper arm and trunk
round the forearm and trunk
round the wrist and thighs

Transport by stretcher.

If a fracture of the radius or ulna or both is suspected, the arm should be supported in a sling and the patient taken to hospital. A similar procedure should be followed for a suspected fracture of the wrist called 'Colles' fracture. This is a common fracture in the winter

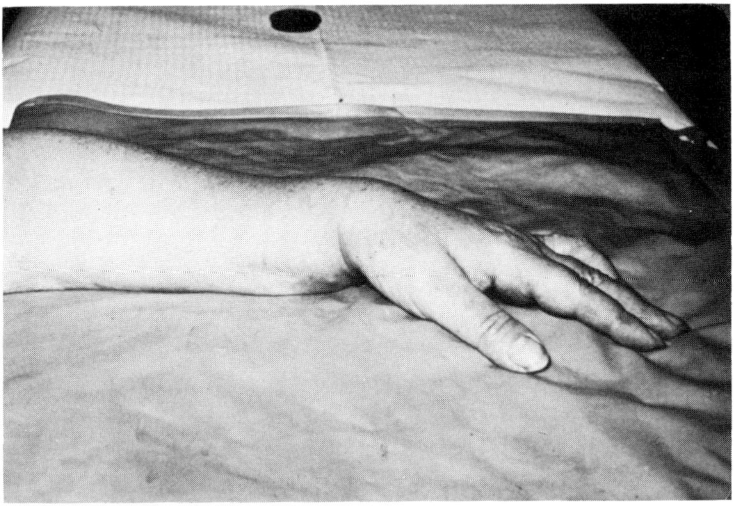

**Fig. 50** 'Dinner fork' deformity of a Colles' fracture.

months when the patient slips on ice or snow and falls forward on to his or her outstretched hand. It is characterised by a 'dinner fork' deformity of the hand (Fig. 50).

### The carpals and metacarpals

Broken fingers can be partially immobilised by strapping them to the uninjured ones and supporting the limb with a triangular bandage. Fractures of the hand and finger bones may be complicated by severe bleeding.

### The ribs

Ribs may be broken by either direct or indirect force. If the force has been direct, there may be a complicated fracture with lung involvement. When there has been indirect force, more than one rib is usually broken because of pressure on both the back and front of the thoracic cage.

The casualty will present with shallow, rapid respiration (in an attempt to limit movement and thereby decrease pain). If the lungs are affected there will be relevant signs and symptoms. When there is a 'sucking' wound of the chest asphyxia can occur if treatment is not given immediately (see Chapter 2).

TREATMENT

*Uncomplicated fracture:* support the upper limb on the affected side with an arm sling. Transport either as a sitting or walking casualty unless otherwise indicated.

*Complicated fracture:* make any 'sucking' wound airtight at once. Support the upper limb with the affected side in an arm sling (Fig. 51a). Lay the casualty down in the semirecumbent position, inclining towards the injured side (Fig. 51b). Support in this position by placing a folded blanket or overcoat lengthwise along the casualty's back and remove to hospital by stretcher as soon as possible.

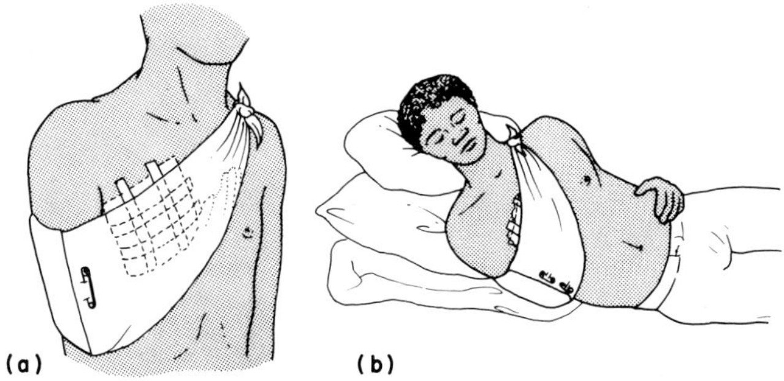


**Fig. 51** Treatment of a complicated fracture of the ribs: (a) first stage and (b) second stage.

## The pelvis

SIGNS AND SYMPTOMS

The casualty will complain of pain in the hips and pelvis made worse by movement. He or she will not be able to stand and may have the desire to pass water frequently. There may be haematuria.

TREATMENT

If a fracture of the pelvis is suspected, great care should be taken to move the patient as little as possible for fear of damaging the pelvic contents (bladder and reproductive organs). The patient should be placed flat with the legs together. Broad bandages should then be tied around the ankles, knees, thighs and hips. Some padding should be placed between the ankles and between the knees. The patient should be discouraged from passing urine. Transport to hospital as soon as possible.

If the journey is likely to be short and smooth, no further first aid is necessary, but if the journey is likely to be delayed or rough and long:

apply 2 broad bandages round the pelvis, overlapping by half, and then control in line with hip joint of the affected side. Tie on the uninjured side

place soft padding between the knees and the ankles; if available padding may be placed between the thighs for greater comfort, apply a figure-of-eight bandage around the ankles and feet and a broad bandage around the knees (Fig. 52).

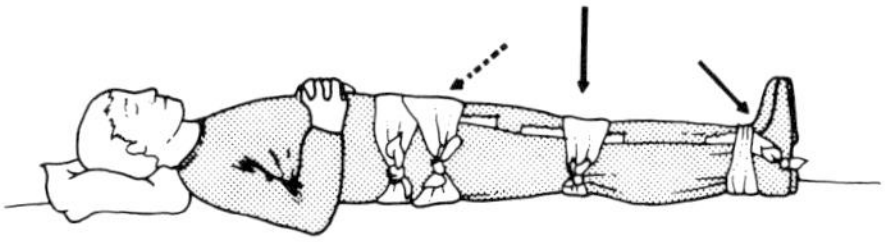

**Fig. 52** Fractured pelvis: preparation for a long or rough journey. The solid arrows indicate essential padding between the knees and ankles. The hatched arrow shows padding which will add to comfort if available.

## The scapula

A fractured scapula is a rare injury and is usually the result of direct force.

TREATMENT

Remove the casualty's coat (and braces as necessary). Place a pad in the axilla of the affected side. Support the arm, with finger-tips pointing to opposite shoulder, in a triangular sling. Give further support by securing the upper limb to the chest with a broad bandage over the sling. Transport to hospital as soon as possible.

## The legs

SIGNS AND SYMPTOMS

A fractured femur is usually easy to diagnose because of the pain, swelling and deformity. The injured leg is often shorter than the other and the foot on the affected side externally rotated. This is not the case, however, if the fracture is impacted: then the bone ends are forced into each other. If an old person who has fallen complains of pain in the hip, he or she should be considered to have fractured the neck of a femur, until diagnosed otherwise.

TREATMENT

Steady and support the injured limb. Bring the sound leg gently to the side of the injured one, and tie limbs together.

When splints are available:

For a fractured tibia and fibula (Fig. 53a):

Apply a well-padded splint between the limbs, extending from the top of the thigh to the foot.

Secure by tying together with broad bandages:

- the ankles and feet with figure-of-eight bandage
- the knees
- the legs
- the thighs
- below the fracture (floater bandage)

Arrange for casualty to be taken to hospital.

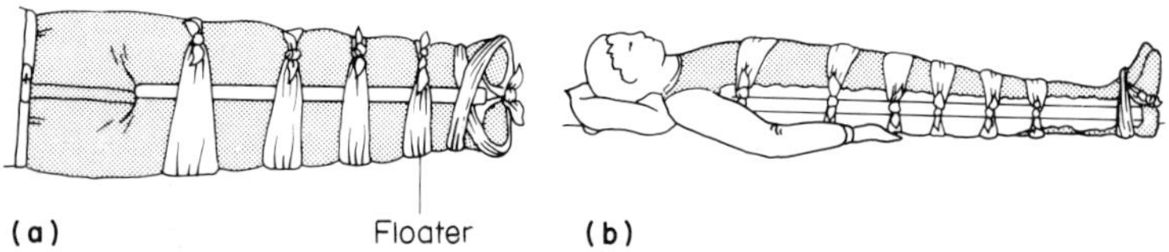


**Fig. 53** Immobilisation of a fractured leg involving (a) the tibia and fibula and (b) the femur.

For a fractured femur (Fig. 53b):

Apply a well-padded splint between the legs and an additional long padded splint to the affected side, extending from the axilla to the foot.

Immobilise with 7 bandages; 5 as previously described for treatment of a fractured tibia and fibula and others around the chest (just below the axillae) and the pelvis.
Arrange transport to hospital as soon as possible.

### The patella

A fractured patella (knee cap) may be the result of muscular action or direct force. A fracture of the patella, tibia or fibula or both (Fig. 54) should be splinted before transport to hospital by using a piece of wood from ankle to thigh. Place soft padding under the ankle to raise the heel off the splint (Fig. 55). The leg should be slightly raised to prevent swelling.

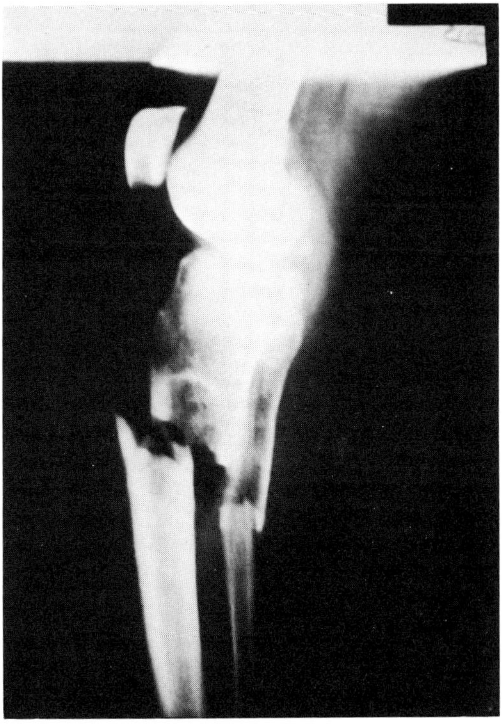

**Fig. 54** X-ray showing a compound fracture of the tibia and fibula.

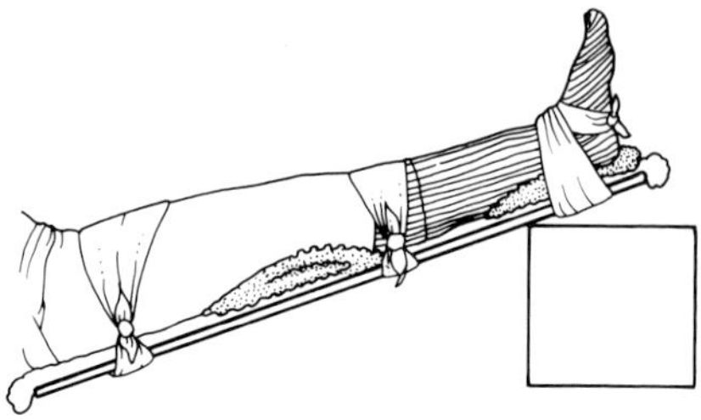

**Fig. 55** Treatment for a fractured patella.

## The ankle

Fractures and sprains of the ankle are often difficult to distinguish. If there is any doubt the patient should be treated as though he or she has a fracture and transported to the hospital for X-ray examination. The most comfortable splint for this purpose is L-shaped and goes along the sole of the patient's foot and up the back of the leg.

TREATMENT

Secure the splint by applying 3 bandages:

- figure-of-eight around the ankle and foot
- broad bandage around the thigh
- broad bandage around the lower leg

Transport with the injured limb in the raised position.

## The tarsals and metatarsals

A foot is crushed usually by a heavy weight dropping on or passing over it. A fracture should be suspected when there is swelling, pain and loss of power.

TREATMENT

Remove shoe, boot, sock or stocking, cutting them off if necessary. Treat any wound present. Apply a well-padded splint to the side of the foot reaching from the heel to the toes. Secure the splint with a figure-of-eight bandage by:

- placing the centre of a broad bandage on the side of the foot
- crossing the ends over the instep and carrying them to the back of the ankle
- crossing them again and bringing them to the front of the ankle
- crossing them once more and passing them under the sole

tying off over the splint

Raise and support the foot in a comfortable position and transfer to hospital.

## OTHER TYPES OF MUSCULOSKELETAL TRAUMA

### Spinal injury

A spinal injury calls for the utmost care when handling the casualty, otherwise the spinal cord may be permanently damaged, causing life-long disability.

Fracture of the spine should always be suspected in all cases in which there is a history of accidental injury to the vertebral column and the victim complains of pain in the back. It may be complicated by injury to the spinal cord, causing complete or partial loss of power or sensation or both below the waist or site of injury. It may result directly from:

A fall from a height and on to the back or across a bar or wall.

A fall of a heavy weight across the casualty's back.

Or from indirect force such as:

A heavy fall on to the feet or buttocks.

A fall on to the head from a height (as in diving).

Overextension or whiplash of the spine (as in a motor car crash).

Even when there is no apparent loss of power or sensation, handle the patient with great care.

#### TREATMENT

Warn the patient to remain still.

If not in a dangerous place, do not move the casualty until you have other skilled help.

Take measures to prevent shock.

In an unconscious patient, the fact that spinal injury has occurred may easily escape consideration. Signs which should arouse suspicion are:

bruising, grazing or other injury to the face or forehead

unusual dryness of the skin of the lower part of the body

complete limpness and lack of spontaneous movement in 2 or all 4 limbs

no reaction to movement of obviously injured limbs

see-saw alteration in movement of the trunk during respiration

Any movement and necessary extension of the neck must be carried out with the greatest care.

SIGNS AND SYMPTOMS

The casualty with paraplegia or tetraplegia, but no other injury will not necessarily show signs of serious shock once the immediate effects of the injury have passed off.

When there is loss of feeling and vasomotor control in the greater part of the body, great diagnostic care is necessary to avoid overlooking other serious injuries.

There may be moderate pallor and the skin may be warm and dry. Signs and symptoms of bleeding must be watched for carefully. Where there are many casualties, the victim with spinal injury and nothing more, need not be given priority transport. Patients with severe haemorrhage, large wounds, deepening unconsciousness, or serious injury of the chest should have priority.

## Management of serious injuries of the back

The main objectives are:

- to protect the spinal cord and nerves
- to provide comfort
- to arrange prompt medical attention

If conscious, the patient should be asked about numbness, weakness, and paralysis as well as pain and injuries apart from those relating to the back. If the casualty is unable to move his or her limbs they should be examined for injury but very carefully, because there will be no pain to warn the patient or first-aider of other fractures. Wounds, swelling, irregularity and deformity must all be looked for, and any injuries found or suspected, treated.

If the patient is already on his or her back, a hand should be passed gently underneath to ascertain injury, taking especial care if there is broken glass lying about. If the casualty is able to move his or her spine without complaint or difficulty, this test can be of great value in diagnosis; the casualty is unlikely to be in danger.

It must be emphasised that casualties should only be asked if they can move. They should not be instructed to move and they must not be made to move.

If the patient is unconscious or shocked or both, very careful examination is essential.

**Preparation for transit to hospital**

The general rule for handling patients with broken bones is that they must be prevented, as far as possible, from causing the bones to move on each other. This is most important in instances of spinal injury. If the patient is conscious, the muscles will splint the injury to some extent and he or she will complain of pain in the injured area. These are safeguards to a degree. If the patient is unconscious, even greater care must be exercised.

A comfortable position need not be altered unless safety or other injuries dictate it; all positions can be and are used when nursing paraplegic patients.

Whilst distorted limbs may be straightened gently after they have been examined for signs of injury, deformities of the spine must never be. The patient's original position should be supported by pads and pillows, and if it has to be altered, the spine must be moved in one piece, keeping the head, shoulders and pelvis in the same relative positions.

The nurse should coordinate the operation, making sure that each helper is clear about what to do. The patient should then be wrapped in a blanket and tied to a board for transportation to hospital. If a spinal or neurosurgical unit is close then efforts should be made to take the patient there.

Even if only a short journey is contemplated, precautions must be taken to avoid pressure on insensitive skin; the first stage of pressure sores occurs within an hour or two of injury.

**Prevention of pressure sores immediately after injury**

Place the patient on a firm, smooth supporting surface.

- Smooth any wrinkled crumpled clothing or blankets.
- Remove hard objects (such as coins and keys in back pockets) from under the patient.
- Fill in natural hollows of the body with pads, maintaining the adopted position.
- Support the head with pads.
- Protect bony prominences from pressure. Place pads under the calves if the patient is on his or her back, or between the knees and feet if lying on his or her side.
- Place pads gently under the hips.
- Loosen constrictions such as straps or shoe laces.

If several hours elapse before arrival in hospital, the patient's position must be changed every 2 hours. The legs should be looked after by one person, shoulders and pelvis by a second, and if the cervical vertebrae are injured, the head by a third. Readjustment of pads in the new position is essential.

If the patient has a broken leg also, it is often better to leave it without splints, but if they are used, they must be very carefully padded and the uninjured as well as the injured leg protected from any pressure which may be caused by splints and knotted bandages.

## Dislocations

Joints most frequently dislocated are those of the shoulder, elbow, thumb, fingers and lower jaw.

A dislocation occurs when the bone (or bones) are displaced from its normal point of articulation.

### SIGNS AND SYMPTOMS

The sufferer experiences severe pain which will prevent movement of the affected part. When compared with the uninjured side, the first-aider will see that there is deformity. There may also be local swelling if there is bleeding into the joint.

### TREATMENT

The nurse should not attempt to put the dislocated bone back. The joint should be immobilised in the most comfortable position and, if the pain is severe, treat the patient for shock. Ice packs will reduce bleeding into the joint space and may also help to relieve the pain.

The patient should be given nothing to drink as he or she may need an anaesthetic before the dislocation is reduced in hospital or surgery.

## Subluxations

A subluxation is a dislocation that returns to its normal place of articulation spontaneously. Subluxations are often difficult to diagnose but the description that the patient gives as to what happened usually helps. The patient should be referred to hospital for X-ray examination. If the joint capsule has been damaged, treatment may be required to immobilise the joint while healing takes place.

## Sprains

A sprain is the tearing, but not complete rupture, of joint ligaments, muscles or joint capsules. It occurs when the joint is forced to go beyond its normal range of movement. It is sometimes difficult to distinguish between a sprain and a fracture and if this is the case, the patient should be treated for a fracture.

### SIGNS AND SYMPTOMS

The patient will complain of pain, particularly when the joint is put through its full range of movement and swelling. Some hours later the area will become discoloured.

### TREATMENT

The first-aider should prevent the casualty from putting weight on the joint. The limb should be raised. A cold compress may be applied and held in position with an elastic bandage. The patient should receive medical aid from his or her own doctor.

## Torn ligament

Where a ligament has been ruptured, the joint concerned is usually unstable. It can be completely or partially dislocated depending which joint is involved. There may also be local pain, tenderness and swelling. The latter may be masked by muscle spasm for a short while after injury.

Gross injury of the ankle is easy to recognise by swelling, deformity and pain. It is difficult, sometimes, to differentiate between sprains and minor fractures. Severe sprains or torn ligaments can be very painful and simulate a fractured ankle. Conversely, there is a danger of diagnosing a fracture as a sprain. Sometimes a positive diagnosis can be made only by X-ray examination, but if the casualty can walk, it is probable that he or she does not have a serious fracture.

TREATMENT

First aid treatment consists of firm support of the ankle by bandaging. This will control swelling and assist weight-bearing.

## Strains

A strain occurs when a muscle or ligament is over-stretched or fatigued. There is no tearing and no swelling. The two commonest causes are athletic sports and lifting a heavy object. The treatment is the same as for a sprain. The injured muscle should be rested until recovery has taken place and it is no longer painful.

## Contusions

Contusions are commonly known as bruises and occur as the result of a direct blow causing capillary damage and bleeding into the soft tissues. Discolouration usually appears several hours later although sometimes it is apparent immediately. Contusions are frequently neglected although pain, swelling and discolouration can often be dramatically reduced by the use of cold compresses and by elevation.

## Head, neck and facial injuries

Injuries affecting this area must be considered life-threatening particularly if the airway is compromised or the brain is damaged. Correct treatment must begin at the scene of the injury, not only to preserve life but also the patient's sight, hearing and appearance.

Although some theoretical explanation is given here, the student is recommended to review the relevant system.

### Craniocerebral injuries

In first aid teaching and practice, particular emphasis is laid upon cerebral compression as a sequel of head injury. This can occur with, or without, fracture.

Any of the meningeal blood vessels may be torn and bleeding. This occurs either between the skull and the dura mater (extradural) or deep to it (subdural). These types of intracranial haemorrhage can occur separately or in various combinations but as far as first aid is concerned, treatment does not vary.

Hypoxic hypoxia occurs frequently and can be dealt with adequately by a first-aider in most instances. The danger is that often it is not recognised or is ignored.

Anaemic hypoxia can be missed also. The head injury patient does not always present with the signs and symptoms of shock. If these exist, a search should be made for other injuries causing serious bleeding. Whether or not these are found, the urgency appropriate to the head injury is increased if shock is present. The reduced oxygen supply that accompanies oligaemic shock may tip the balance against the recovery of the brain. Immediate resuscitation is vital.

**The brain**

Brain tissue is extremely sensitive and a blow to the head with no observable brain damage can lead to sudden loss of consciousness. This is thought to be due to a sudden shock wave being sent through the cerebral hemispheres and is called concussion.

Injury to the brain tissue causes swelling and haemorrhage just as in any other part of the body. Due to the small amount of space within the skull, the pressure can build up quickly leading to loss of function. This so-called raised intracranial pressure must be relieved as quickly as possible or permanent damage may result.

The central nervous system has no capacity to repair itself. Any damage to the nervous tissue is permanent. The first-aider must therefore be extremely careful not to cause any further injury by improper lifting or positioning of the patient who should be transported to hospital with the greatest speed.

**The skull**

Fractures of the skull are not necessarily important in themselves. They become so when the bone is depressed, causing damage to the brain beneath, or when there is damage to the blood vessels leading to intracerebral haemorrhage and subsequent compression of the brain. An uncomplicated skull fracture is either linear or stellate and will heal spontaneously without treatment (Fig. 56). The patient may, of course, need other treatment for a lacerated scalp or concussion. Fractures of the base of the skull are difficult to detect. They may manifest themselves with the leakage of blood or cerebrospinal fluid or both from the nose or the ear. The appearance of unexplained bruising around both

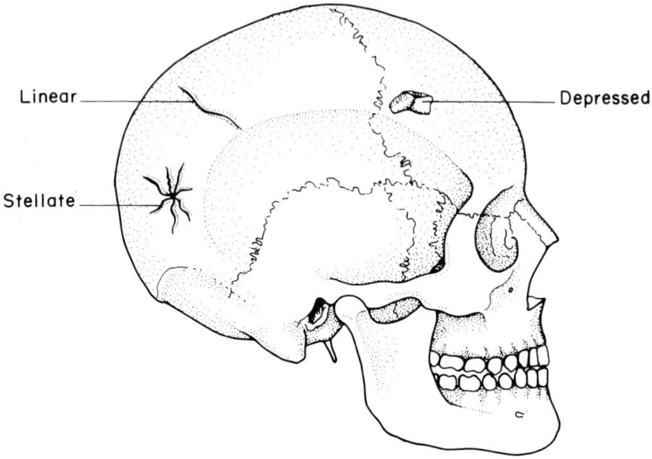


**Fig. 56** Types of skull fracture.

eyes should alert the nurse that a fracture of the base of the skull is a possibility.

**Cerebral haemorrhages**

These fall into three categories:

**1** An extradural haematoma occurs when the small vessels between the skull and the dura are damaged and a haematoma develops between them. It is self-perpetuating because as the clot enlarges, further separation occurs and more vessels are damaged. The development is slow and the level of consciousness deteriorates gradually. The site of the haematoma is beneath the fracture site.

**2** A subdural haematoma develops between the dura and the vascular arachnoid. It can be of a very rapid onset. It is commonly the diagnosis when a patient who is conscious soon after the injury rapidly becomes unconscious 1 to 2 hours later.

**3** Subarachnoid haemorrhage usually occurs following trauma only when there is underlying blood vessel disease such as atheroma or aneurysm. It occurs suddenly and may also be associated with a blood clot in the brain itself.

**Contrecoup injury**

When the head is struck, the skull moves first, and then the brain, floating within it, gathers momentum. The movement of the skull is then halted rapidly by the limitations of the structures joining it to the rest of the body. The brain by this time is accelerating and the two are set on a collision course. This impact of the brain against the inside of the skull can cause damage worse than that at the point of impact. The possibility of signs of cerebral oedema and haemorrhage should therefore be considered, on either side.

TREATMENT

It cannot be overstated that the two main points to remember in the management of a patient with brain damage is the maintenance of adequate respirations and secondly the avoidance of any action that could make the condition worse. A build-up of carbon dioxide in the blood will increase cerebral oedema in an already damaged brain causing further damage which could be permanent.

If the brain is visible outside the wound, it should not be cleaned and no pressure should be applied. A light gauze dressing held in place by a loose bandage is the best first aid treatment. If it is possible to elevate the top part of the patient's body, this should be done, but the head should not be placed on a pillow as this could cause further damage to the spinal cord or block the airway.

Even though the patient may be conscious and alert when she or he arrives on the scene, the first-aider should continue to assess the patient carefully as deterioration can be dramatic and sudden. The first-aider should be prepared to instigate resuscitative measures at any time. A close watch should be made of the casualty's pupils. A dilated pupil reacting sluggishly to light is a cardinal sign of rising pressure on that side of the brain. The pulse too must be carefully monitored as a bradycardia is also an indication of raised intracranial pressure. (Should a sphygmomanometer be available an associated elevation of the blood pressure would be found.)

Abnormal electrical activity in the brain following an injury could lead to the patient having a seizure. Should this occur the patient must be prevented from injuring him or herself, but should not be restrained. The nurse must remember that apnoea (lack of respiration) during the tonic or rigid stage of the fit is due to muscle spasm and not to an obstructed airway. On no account should the first-aider put her or his fingers into the patient's mouth while a seizure is taking place.

If, after due consideration, there appears to be no damage to the cervical spine, the patient may be gently positioned in the recovery position (Fig. 32, page 51). When making this decision, the nurse should take care to place the patient on the appropriate side. If there is any leakage from one ear, that side should be placed downwards so that drainage can continue freely. If a portion of brain is protruding through a break in the skull on no account should the patient be placed so that there is pressure on this area, as this could cause death.

### The facial bones

There are 18 bones in the face. All of them are fixed, apart from the mandible or lower jaw, which articulates with the temporal bone on each side. Some of these bones are more prominent than others and so are more susceptible to damage.

#### SIGNS AND SYMPTOMS

Fractures of the facial bones are almost always associated with bleeding from the nose and mouth and severe swelling which could obstruct the airway.

#### TREATMENT

Assessment and care of the patient following injury to the head and neck region is vital to their survival. The aim of treatment is to:

preserve life
maintain function
restore appearance

These injuries often look dramatic and the first-aider needs to remember that although facial lacerations often bleed briskly they are rarely life-threatening. She or he should not be distracted by them.

Initially a quick but accurate evaluation is required. On arrival at the scene of an accident, the nurse should make the following checks on each casualty:

signs of any obstruction to the airway
serious bleeding that could be life-threatening
the level of consciousness

The consciousness level should be assessed and recorded, in case of any change in the future. For example, a patient may be knocked unconscious and quickly become fully alert. Conversely, the level of consciousness may deteriorate gradually. Specific terms should be used to describe the conscious level. These include—alert; confused; drowsy; unconscious but responding to pain; and deeply unconscious with no response.

A patient who is conscious should be questioned as to who and where he or she is and the approximate date and time. The nurse should also establish the site of any pain the patient has, and whether or not there is any tingling, numbness or loss of sensation.

Evaluating an unconscious patient is much more difficult. It should be remembered that if the injury was sufficient to render the patient unconscious, there may well be underlying brain or spinal cord damage. The patient should be handled very carefully indeed. Information may be sought from any observers who are around.

CHAPTER 6

# Trauma III: Bomb Blast Injuries and Bullet Wounds

In many countries societal violence is becoming a growing problem and nurses are increasingly being confronted with the care of victims of bombs and bullets.

In a climate of civil unrest and sudden violence, bomb explosions or shoot-outs between opposing factions can lead to the possibility of many people being wounded and arriving simultaneously at hospital. Such incidents would indicate serious unrest in the community and are likely to be repeated. Management in hospital often involves disaster drill which places on nursing staff a heavy burden of responsibility. It is essential that the disaster plan is frequently reviewed and kept up-to-date, that nursing staff are familiar with it and are prepared to put the plan into action at any time. The efficiency of such a plan is dependent on the competence of personnel involved. Effective nursing practice requires a breadth of knowledge in the nurse dealing with emergencies, which is not found in traditional nursing practice. Nurses are constantly having to broaden their knowledge and increase their level of competence to enable them to expand and extend their role in patient care.

## BOMB BLAST INJURIES

Because of the gross mutilation which may be produced by an explosion, the bomb is probably the most feared of all weapons available today.

A bomb consists of an explosive material enclosed in a container of some sort, with a detonator to set off the explosion and perhaps a timing device. When a bomb explodes, enormous volumes of gases are produced and energy is dissipated radially. A high pressure wave at high velocity spreads outwards followed by a negative pressure phase.

The terrorist bomb differs from the wartime bomb in that it is nearly always delivered by hand or by motor vehicle. Some of these bombs are made with the intention of injuring one victim or a small group of victims, for example, letter bombs, booby traps, anti-personnel bombs. When a bomb of 2·5 to 3 kg explodes in an enclosed space, as in a room, casualties will be caused by the blast itself, by flying debris and perhaps by falling masonry. A car bomb contains a much larger charge, for example, 230 kg, and when this explodes without warning, those closest may be blown to pieces by the force of the blast or may suffer serious mutilating injuries, while the majority of casualties will suffer relatively minor injuries from flying debris. Others in the vicinity of the blast may not sustain any physical injury but suffer tremendous nervous shock from the explosion and perhaps from witnessing the gross trauma sustained by other people.

Flying debris may include fragments of bomb casing which, close to the bomb, may behave like high velocity missiles. Because of irregularity in their shape, however, they are slowed down in air and also on passage through clothing and tissues. Other debris may include metal, wood, stones, or any object picked up from the environment by the blast. One of the greatest dangers is from flying glass which can inflict horrific injuries.

The blast effect may also produce damage to the walls of hollow organs, commonly the middle ear, lungs and gastrointestinal tract.

**Disaster drill**

When a bomb explodes in a crowded area there is the possibility of many being wounded and arriving simultaneously at the hospital. Management of bomb explosions often involves disaster drill and it is vital that nursing staff are familiar with this so that it may be implemented immediately. The disaster can be dealt with most effectively when manned by staff who know the department well, but other staff can assist with observations, transfer of patients and in coping with shocked patients and relatives.

Minor cases should be treated as expeditiously as possible and nurses should be allocated to ensure that these are dealt with along with the 'normal' casualties, while others are looking after the more seriously injured. Other staff who have come to offer help, should leave the department if they are not required, as masses of people milling around leads to increased confusion and the possibility of error.

The best place for the care of serious casualties is the normal surgical ward and it would seem better to set up a special area to which the more able patients can be transferred, while staff of surgical wards can get on with caring for those badly injured in their familiar surroundings.

One important aspect of dealing with such a disaster is that of keeping the media informed and someone fairly senior from the administrative staff should take this responsibility. Adequate documentation of cases with a copy for the information centre is vital and the centre should coordinate all information as it is received.

**Effects on the human body**

Despite the bizarre combinations of injuries which may result from bombs, the principles of care are the same as for any patient with multiple injuries. Initial evaluation, resuscitation and stabilisation may determine whether trauma victims survive. The priorities of emergency care can easily be remembered, under the headings A, B and C, that is Airway, Breathing, Circulation. Assessment, initiation of life support measures and management of the injuries must proceed simultaneously and the nurse has a major part to play. Well-defined spheres of medical and nursing practice overlap when nurse and doctor work together to resuscitate a patient. Providing high quality care is more important than who does what, and this implies competence in the provider of care. Nurses working in emergency departments have an obligation to ensure that they are adequately prepared and capable of taking appropriate action where life-saving procedures are required.

The main difference between the management of road traffic accidents and bomb blast injuries is gross tissue damage and wound contamination. Theatre nurses will find themselves fully employed for many hours following a bomb blast as thorough debridement, with careful excision of all dead tissue, is very important. Primary suture is rarely attempted but undertaken later when all divided muscle is seen to be absolutely healthy and uncontaminated. Apparently superficial wounds need to be carefully assessed and explored if there is any doubt, as the underlying wound may be serious. Initial surgical treatment is usually completed in a few hours but a residual volume of surgery may be required in many cases, often up to 2 or more years after the injury.

Persons close to the centre of an explosion may sustain flash burns from the chemical reaction. They are likely to be mainly to the hands and face as clothing provides protection from flash. Burns may also be caused by burning clothing or by the building being set on fire. Nurses play a major part in the care of these patients who usually require long periods of hospitalisation, often involving skin grafting and plastic surgery.

One common and immediate effect of bomb blast is damage to ears; the eardrum may be perforated, producing tinnitus and sensorineural deafness. Patients may not realise they are totally deaf, nor, indeed, may those looking after them, so it is vital that nurses are aware of the possibility of this effect when caring for bomb blast victims.

Damage to the lungs from blast effect may not appear immediately, and close observation is important for the early detection of signs of respiratory failure. While this condition may be seen in only a small proportion of bomb blast victims, it can be present in those who have sustained no other injury. Massive lung haemorrhage and oedema are common post mortem findings in those killed by bombs.

## GUNSHOT WOUNDS

The capacity of a missile to injure depends on the amount of energy it contains and the transfer of that energy. The velocity of the missile is of more importance than the mass. A bullet fired from a high velocity weapon passes through the body, not only destroying structures in its path but creating a zone of cavitation around it. Shock waves damage the tissues directly and as the cavity collapses, contaminated particles are sucked in via the entrance and exit wounds. This combination of dead tissue and contamination produces ideal conditions for clostridial infections with a high risk of gas gangrene. Low velocity bullets produce a track roughly the size of the missile and the cavitation effect is minimal or absent. These bullets are usually arrested in the tissues and are often deflected by important structures during their passage. A bullet which does not exit from the body may not travel in a straight line and its final location may be an unexpected one.

When a shotgun is used, many small particles of lead shot are projected and the extent of the damage depends on the distance of the body from the gun muzzle. Close range injuries cause extensive soft tissue damage while a discharge from a sawn-off shotgun can penetrate the thorax or abdomen. Discharges at greater distances may leave numerous metallic pellets in the subcutaneous tissues, but are unlikely to produce serious injury unless an eye is struck or a major artery penetrated. The excision of large masses of scattered pellets is not possible and most will do no harm if left alone. Patients tend to be upset and fearful of such foreign bodies and need a great deal of understanding and reassurance.

**Effects on the human body**

When a patient who has been shot is admitted to hospital, it is important to completely undress him or her in order to search for additional wounds and injuries. The missile track can usually be determined by noting entrance and exit wounds and assuming a straight line course. Entrance wounds are usually surprisingly small and round and may show discoloration of the surrounding skin. Exit wounds tend to be irregular in shape (Fig. 57). If no exit wound is found retained bullets must be located by X-ray. When bone is struck by a bullet, it will probably shatter, the bullet will be deflected and pieces of bone may become secondary missiles, thus producing increased tissue damage and perhaps a large exit wound. The aim of wound cleansing is to remove debris and to control infection without causing further damage to injured tissue.

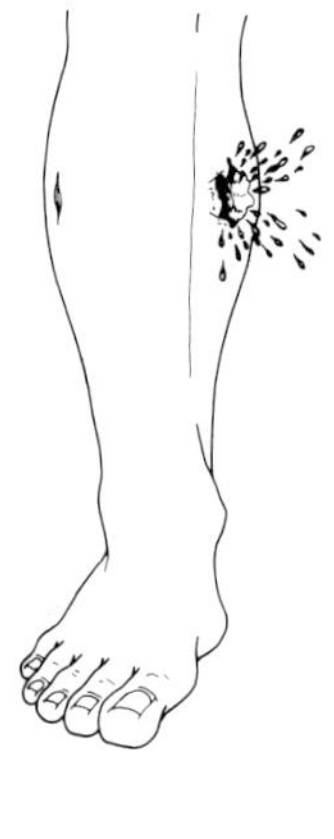

**Fig. 57** Gunshot wound showing a small entry and a larger exit.

*Chest*

Penetrating chest wounds often result in a sucking wound, which must be sealed immediately. Insertion of chest drains and constant observation of blood loss is vital as haemothorax is a common result of such injury. The possibility of cardiac tamponade must also be kept in mind. Nurses need to be aware of the signs of cardiac tamponade, that is hypotension, distended neck veins and distant heart signs. The onset of these signs may be insidious, and immediate surgical intervention is essential if the patient is to survive. Because lung tissue is less dense than other tissues, it has a lower resistance so shock wave is much less and tissue damage is reduced. The possibility of damage to the great vessels must not be overlooked however, and there is a good chance that missiles entering the chest may end up in the neck, head, abdomen or limbs.

*Abdomen*

Initial examination of the patient should detect penetrating abdominal wounds. An evisceration may occur which will require moist saline dressings and the application of a pressure bandage. High velocity missile injury to the abdomen will cause massive shattering of tissues and the mortality rate is high. The spine may also be damaged due to transmission of shock waves.

All abdominal penetrating wounds require surgical exploration, and where the bowel has been penetrated, peritoneal contamination by faecal content is inevitable and nursing care may be arduous and prolonged. Nurses need to be alert to signs and symptoms indicating abscess formation and wound infection.

*Head*

Successful treatment of severe head injuries depends on the speed with which the patient reaches the accident centre, and care provided has a profound effect on the outcome. The initial level of consciousness should not influence management as it is no indication of eventual outcome. There is likely to be a rise in intracranial pressure due to bleeding and oedema and, when necessary, intubation must be performed urgently to allow hyperventilation. The reaction of pupils to light and the patient's response to painful stimuli should be rapidly assessed. Exploratory surgery must be undertaken, clot and bone fragments removed from the bullet track and metallic fragments removed only if readily accessible. Intracranial pressure monitoring should be undertaken and the need for controlled hyperventilation may necessitate the patient's admission to an intensive care unit.

CHAPTER 7

# Obstetric Emergencies

On or off duty, a nurse may have to deal with an emergency in which the woman

is pregnant *or*
is in labour *or*
is giving birth *or*
has just given birth

In all these circumstances, it is essential to remain cool, calm and collected, giving reassurance to the patient and clear concise instructions to those nearby who can help.

## EMERGENCIES IN PREGNANT WOMEN

### Antepartum haemorrhage

Antepartum haemorrhage is bleeding from, or into, the genital tract after the twenty-eighth week of pregnancy and before birth of the child. It can be due to:

abruptio placentae *or*
unavoidable haemorrhage *or*
incidental bleeding

**Abruptio placentae (accidental antepartum haemorrhage)**
In cases of abruptio placentae, the bleeding is due to the premature separation of a normally situated placenta. It may be seen (revealed) or concealed behind the placenta (Fig. 58).

The condition is associated with:

folic acid deficiency *or*
pre-eclampsia or hypertension or both *or*
(following) an attempt to turn the fetus

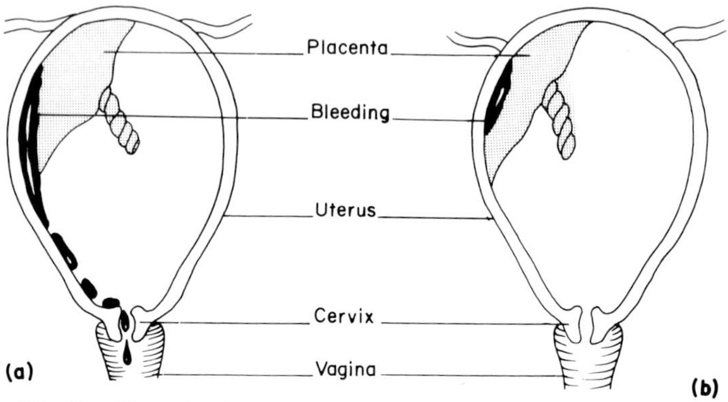


**Fig. 58** Abruptio placentae: (a) revealed and (b) concealed bleeding.

SIGNS AND SYMPTOMS

bleeding from the vagina

abdominal pain

palpable fetus (unless bleeding is totally or partially concealed)

Sometimes there will be:

raised blood pressure

oedema of feet, ankles, pretibial areas of the legs, vulva, sacrum, abdomen, hands and eyelids

protein in the urine

If the bleeding is concealed, or is a combination of revealed and concealed, the patient is likely to complain of continuous pain. Her abdomen will be hard and tender to touch. The fetus will not be palpable. The patient may be in a shocked state (see page 58–62).

TREATMENT

Lay the patient on her side, making her as comfortable as possible.

Reassure her.

Give her nothing by mouth.

Send for medical or midwifery help or the flying squad from the nearest maternity unit.

Remove to hospital.

The patient's blood pressure, pulse rate and colour should be recorded every 10 minutes until she reaches hospital.

During this time, save all urine she passes and all sanitary pads so that the total blood loss may be estimated.

HOSPITAL MANAGEMENT

Management in hospital will consist of resuscitation as necessary, and artificial rupture of the membranes. This will be followed by the setting up of a syntocinon infusion or, if the fetus is still alive, by Caesarean section.

**Placenta praevia (unavoidable antepartum haemorrhage)**

In instances of placenta praevia the bleeding is due to partial separation of the placenta with siting partly or completely in the lower uterine segment (Fig. 59).

SIGNS AND SYMPTOMS

Bleeding from the vagina (even when resting) is often the only sign.

There is no abdominal pain, no signs or symptoms of shock and no abdominal tenderness. The fetus may be felt with ease.

TREATMENT

Treatment is the same as that previously described for abruptio placentae.

HOSPITAL MANAGEMENT

Management in hospital will include resuscitation as necessary. The pregnancy will be prolonged until the thirty-eighth week if possible and then, depending upon the site of the placenta, membranes will be ruptured artificially (if type I or type II) or Caesarean section will be performed (if type III or type IV).

**Incidental bleeding**

Bleeding is associated here with certain conditions of the cervix or vagina. The cause is likely to be:

cervical erosion *or*
cervical polyp *or*
cervical fibroid *or*
carcinoma of the cervix *or*
an infection of the vagina

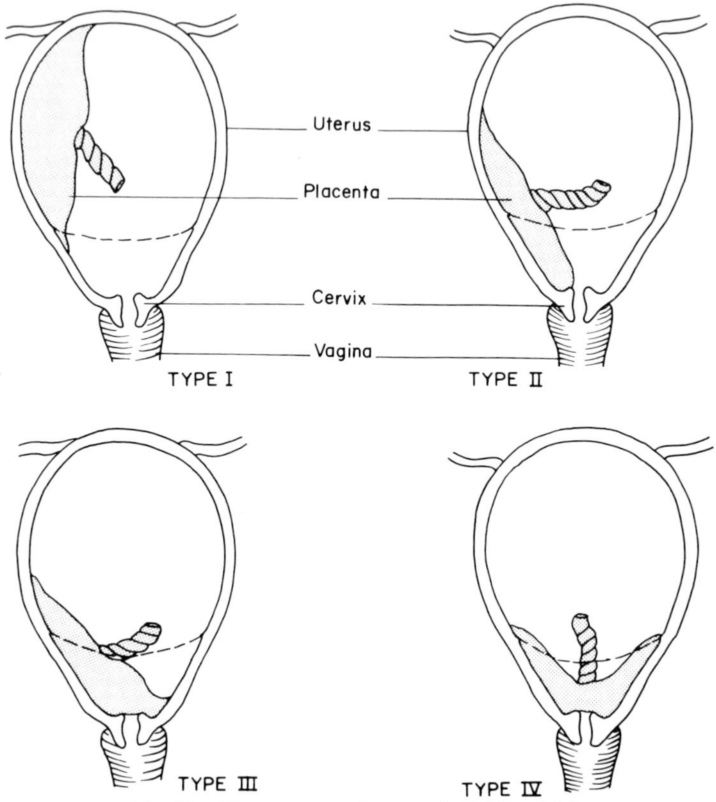


**Fig. 59** Placenta praevia: types I, II, III and IV.

SIGNS AND SYMPTOMS

Again, bleeding from the vagina may be the only sign. There are no signs or symptoms of shock and the fetus is easily palpable.

TREATMENT

Treatment is the same as that previously described for abruptio placentae.

HOSPITAL MANAGEMENT

Management in hospital will include diagnosis and, whenever possible, treatment of the cause.

## Pre-eclampsia

Pre-eclampsia is a condition peculiar to pregnancy. The cause is unknown. It may occur any time after the twenty-eighth week of pregnancy and is characterised by:

raised blood pressure
oedema (Fig. 60) *and*
protein in the urine

The patient should be referred to her general practitioner if these three cardinal signs appear.

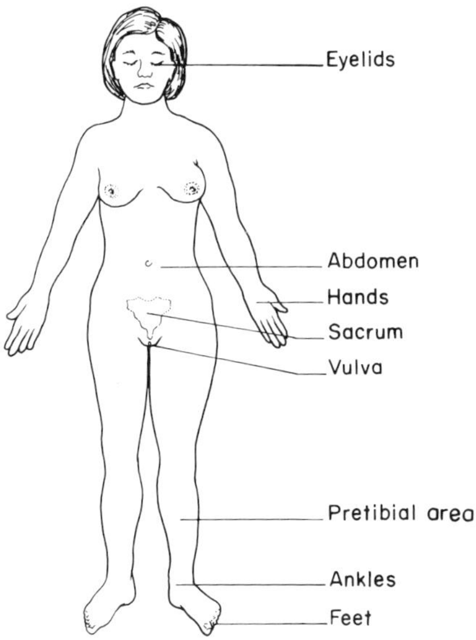


**Fig. 60** Possible sites for oedema.

SERIOUS SIGNS AND SYMPTOMS

Marked rise in blood pressure from 140/90 to 160/100 or over.
Increased oedema.

An increase in the amount of protein in the urine (this may rise up to 12 g per litre).
Severe frontal headaches (rather like those associated with migraine).
Visual disturbances (flashing lights or spots before the eyes).
Vomiting and epigastric discomfort.
Diminished urinary output.

These signs and symptoms constitute an emergency situation and eclampsia may develop.

Summon transport to hospital as soon as possible. Fits which occur are of an epileptic type. They may be followed by coma.

TREATMENT

After sending for help in the form of general practitioner, midwife or flying squad:

Place the patient in a lateral or semiprone position.
Remove her dentures, hairpins and the like.
Loosen her clothing around the neck and waist.
Prevent self injury (this includes keeping the tongue forward and preventing the patient from biting it).
Keep the patient quiet (if possible, in an unoccupied room which has just enough light for observation).
Observe and record every 30 minutes:
 blood pressure
 pulse
 colour
Give nothing by mouth.
Transfer to hospital under sedation and with an escort.

HOSPITAL MANAGEMENT

If the patient's condition does not improve within 36 hours, the pregnancy will be terminated by Caesarean section.

If the patient's condition does improve satisfactorily, the pregnancy may be allowed to continue until the thirty-seventh week, when labour will be induced.

## Eclampsia

Eclampsia is a condition which is also peculiar to pregnancy. It is characterised by convulsions and coma. It may occur during pregnancy or during labour or up to 12 hours after delivery.

SIGNS AND SYMPTOMS

Blood pressure 140/90 or above.
Obvious oedema of face vulva and other areas (Fig. 60).
Protein in the urine.
Intense frontal headache.
Visual disturbances.
Epigastric pain.
Vomiting.

It must be remembered, however, that all these warning signs and symptoms may be absent and a convulsion occur without them. There are four stages to this type of fit:

**Stage 1** The patient becomes very restless, her face twitches and her eyes roll.
**Stage 2** The whole body becomes rigid, respirations cease and severe cyanosis develops. Her teeth will be clenched and her eyes staring.
**Stage 3** The body gives violent jerky movements. The patient's face becomes congested and distorted. She may froth at the mouth. As the convulsive movements subside, the patient goes into:
**Stage 4** Coma. This may last for minutes or for hours.

TREATMENT

After summoning expert help, the main aim of the first-aider is to prevent the patient from injuring herself and:

keep the patient's airway clear by turning the patient on to her right side
remove any dentures and hairpins and loosen any restricting garments (especially at waist, neck and across her chest)
prevent other injury to herself (for example, move furniture out of reach)
observe and record every 15 minutes:
pulse and respiration rates
colour and temperature

take blood pressure every 15 minutes
note how long the fit lasts
give oxygen by mask when the fit is over

If the fit occurs during pregnancy, it is important to be alert for the onset of labour.

SIGNS AND SYMPTOMS

Rhythmic, regular, painful uterine contractions.
The passage of a plug of mucus from the vagina (this may be blood stained).
The cervix begins to dilate.

HOSPITAL MANAGEMENT

Management in hospital is aimed primarily to prevent another fit from occurring and the administration of heavy sedation is essential to this end. Intravenous valium or apresoline may be given to reduce the blood pressure. There are then three alternatives:

spontaneous labour and delivery by low forceps
induction of labour by the administration of syntocinon *or*
Caesarean section

The last is most often thought to be advisable.

In order to prevent further fits, the patient will be well sedated for 48 hours after delivery.

Good nursing is an essential part of the treatment of this emergency.

## Premature rupture of the membranes

Generally, the membranes break at the beginning of labour. When they rupture before the start of labour it is called premature rupture of the membranes.

SIGNS AND SYMPTOMS

The only sign is likely to be watery loss from the vagina (forewater). This may be a sudden rush of water or a small amount of fluid may drain intermittently (Fig. 61).

TREATMENT

Reassure the patient.

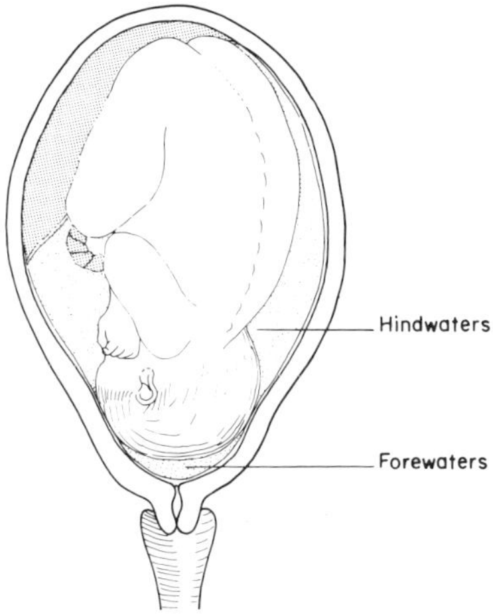


**Fig. 61** Premature rupture of the membranes.

Get her to lie down if possible.

Send for an ambulance to transport her to hospital.

It is important to note both odour and colour of the loss: green fluid is often indicative of fetal distress.

Management in hospital will be mainly a matter of close observation for even if the patient is not in labour, there is always a danger of intra-uterine infection or cord prolapse.

## Cord prolapse

The cord may prolapse after the membranes have ruptured; it may not be seen or it may lie outside the vulva (Fig. 62). It is necessary to send for expert help and an ambulance to take the patient to hospital.

### TREATMENT

Place the patient in the exaggerated Simms left lateral position, inserting 2 pillows under her buttocks to take the pressure of the presenting part of the cord. (If the nurse has experience of performing vaginal examinations, she or he may, with sterile-gloved fingers, manually elevate the presenting part of the cord.)

Emergency treatment for this complication of pregnancy is of

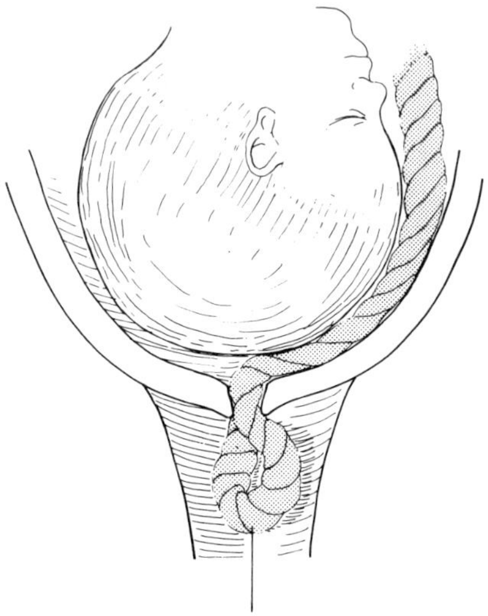


**Fig. 62** Cord prolapse.

extreme urgency. If not dealt with quickly and efficiently the result will be a stillbirth.

HOSPITAL MANAGEMENT

Hospital management will depend on the stage of labour. Those patients who are in the first stage of labour or are not yet in labour, will be delivered by Caesarean section. Those in the second stage, will have an episiotomy performed and a forceps delivery. If the cord is not pulsating, labour will be allowed to continue without interference, but the outcome will be a stillbirth.

## Precipitate labour

Whilst precipitate labour is a comparatively rare occurrence, it usually happens in the most inconvenient places, and at the most inconvenient times. Nurses may well find themselves the only people available to help the mother.

SIGNS AND SYMPTOMS

A few (three or four) rhythmic, regular and painful uterine contractions.

The passage of a plug of mucus.

Dilation of the cervix.

A feeling of having her bowels open (means that the baby is about to be born).

TREATMENT

Explain to the patient what is happening.

Send for expert help or ambulance or both.

Lay the patient flat on her back with support for her head (the equivalent of 2 or 3 pillows).

Loosen any tight restricting garments.

Expose the external genitalia, avoiding overexposure.

**Stages of delivery**

The stages of delivery (shown in Figs. 63–67) include the position of the attendant's hands as the fetal head advances; the position of the attendant's hands when the fetal head is nearly delivered; checking to see that the cord is not around the neck; assisting the delivery of the shoulders and the body; placing the baby on the mother's abdomen and clearing the baby's air passages.

TREATMENT

After delivery:

wrap the baby in a warm blanket

if possible, let the mother hold the baby

do not cut the cord (await the arrival of a midwife or doctor to do this)

**Delivery of the placenta and membranes**

A nurse may well have to manage this last stage of labour. Place a bowl at the vulva and watch carefully the amount of bleeding from the vagina (a 'cat-like' vigilance is needed in order that any excess is noted and dealt with quickly). This should be minimal and between 100 and 200 ml.

The patient will probably say that she feels the pushing. On

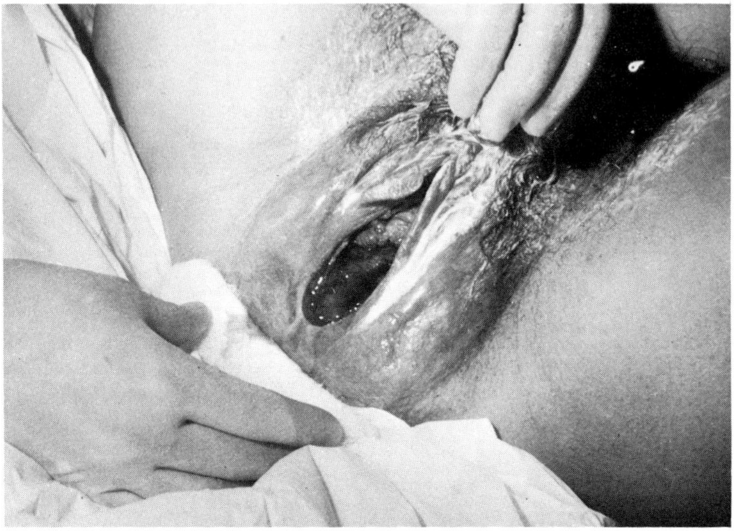

**Fig. 63** The fetal head is advancing—note the position of the attendant's hands.

palpation a round hard mass—often described as being like a cricket ball—may be felt just below the umbilicus. Allow the patient to push and delivery of placenta and membranes (Fig. 68) will probably take place. The average blood loss at this stage is 200–300 ml.

The membranes and placenta should be kept for inspection by the midwife.

Make the mother as comfortable as possible, keeping her and the baby warm until help comes. Give the mother nothing by mouth until the membranes and placenta have been inspected and found to be complete.

During the waiting time, observe every 10–15 minutes:

maternal pulse
colour
bleeding from the vagina
uterus (this should remain hard. If it becomes soft and boggy, gently massage over the fundus until it becomes hard)
blood pressure

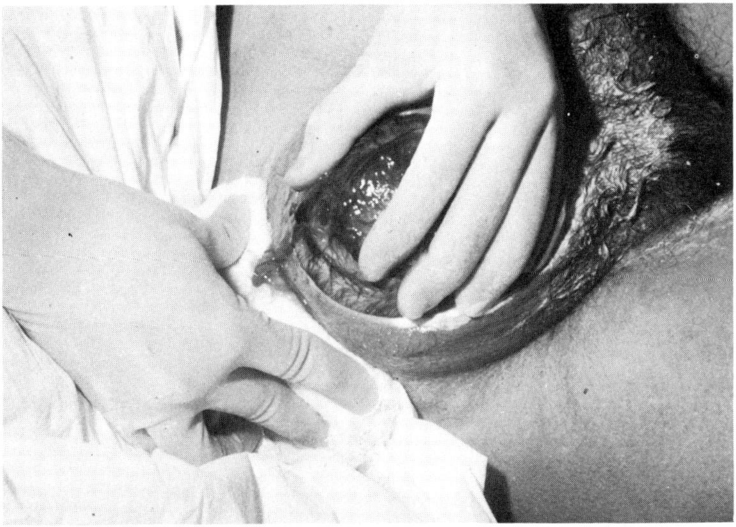

**Fig. 64** The fetal head is nearly delivered—note the position of the attendant's hands and allow the head to deliver slowly.

If the baby shows signs of asphyxia, treat as described on pages 130–1.

Before arrival of the midwife, it is important to give a great deal of reassurance and comfort to the mother who could find the birth both physically and emotionally traumatic.

## Postpartum haemorrhage

Postpartum haemorrhage is bleeding of any amount (usually 600 ml or more) which causes deterioration in the patient's condition after the birth of a baby and within 24 hours of delivery.

It may occur when the placenta and membranes are still *in situ* or after they have been delivered.

TREATMENT

If the placenta is still in the uterus:

Reassure the mother.

Send for expert help.

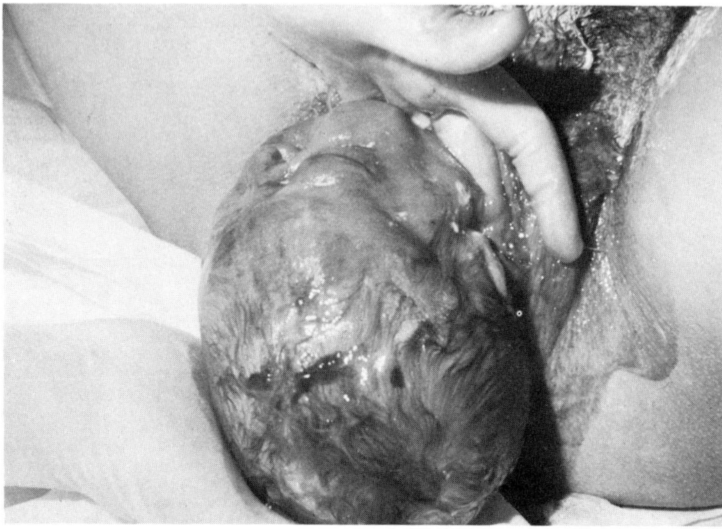

**Fig. 65** Check to see the cord is not around the neck.

Gently palpate the uterus (just below the umbilicus) which will feel soft and boggy.

Place a hand over the fundus of the uterus and gently massage the uterus until it becomes hard (like a cricket ball).

Keep the hand behind and over the fundus and repeat the massage if or when the uterus becomes soft again.

Allow the baby to suckle each breast for 2–3 minutes each side. This stimulates the posterior lobe of the pituitary gland to secrete oxytocin, which causes the uterus to contract.

Give syntometrine (1 ampoule) intramuscularly as soon as this is available.

Give nothing by mouth.

Keep the patient warm.

Observe every 10 minutes or as often as the patient's condition indicates:

maternal pulse

blood pressure (if possible)

colour

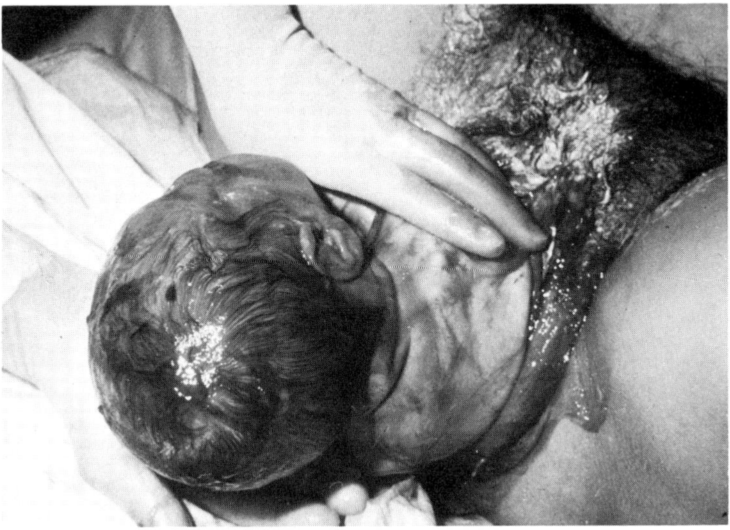

**Fig. 66** Assisting the delivery of the shoulders and the body.

Encourage the patient to pass urine, as a full bladder can be the cause of her relaxed uterus. (Ideally she should be catheterised.)

Keep all sanitary towels, so that the total blood loss can be estimated.

MANAGEMENT

The placenta and membranes may be delivered by controlled cord traction, or they may have to be removed manually later in hospital when the patient's condition has improved.

When post partum haemorrhage occurs after the placenta and membranes have been delivered, the emergency treatment is the same as that described for when the placenta is still in utero.

### Traumatic postpartum haemorrhage

Bleeding is from a tear of the cervix, vagina or the perineal body.

SIGNS AND SYMPTOMS

Excessive bleeding from the vagina.

Palpable round hard uterus.

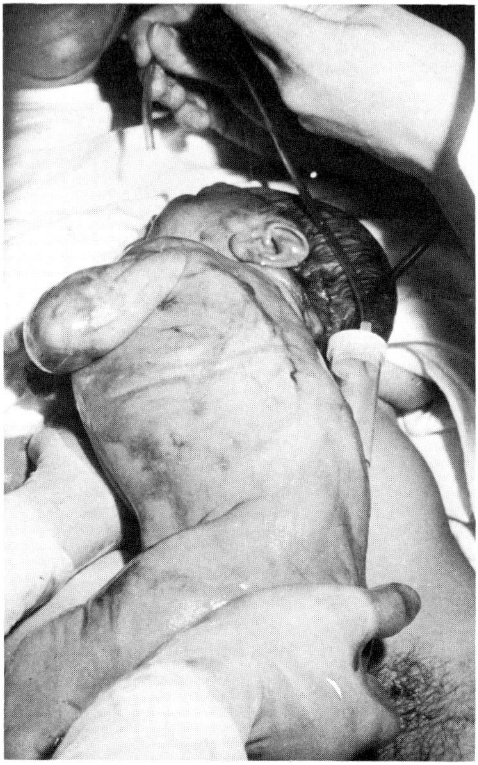

**Fig. 67** Place the baby on the mother's abdomen and clear the air passages.

TREATMENT

Send for expert help as suturing of the laceration will be required.

Reassure the patient and keep her warm.

Apply pressure to the site with a sterile pad.

Observe and record:

- pulse every 10 minutes
- loss of blood
- colour
- blood pressure

Give nothing by mouth.

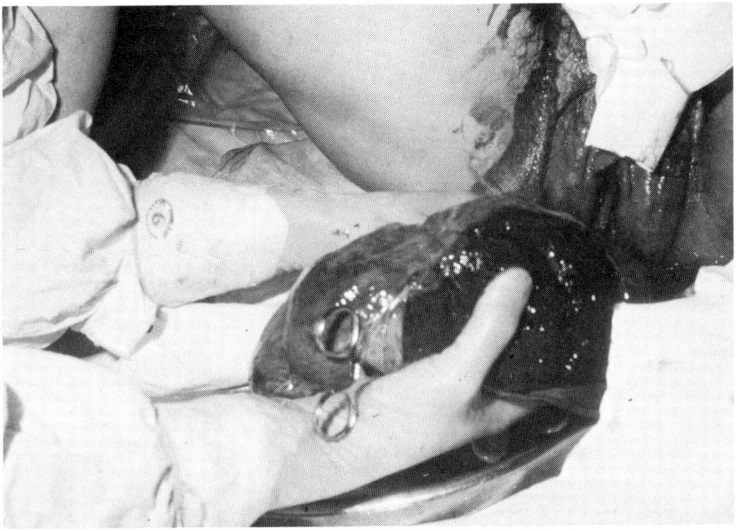

**Fig. 68** Delivery of the placenta and membranes.

*Sudden collapse*

Sudden collapse can occur in patients with traumatic postpartum haemorrhage. Vigilant care is vital.

SIGNS AND SYMPTOMS

Thready, soft pulse of a rate 70–120 per minute.
Fall in blood pressure.
Pallor.
Cold, clammy skin.
Rapid irregular respirations.

TREATMENT

Treatment is as previously described for postpartum haemorrhage.

*In addition:*

elevate the patient's feet and legs (lift up the foot of her bed or couch with blocks of wood if appropriate)
ensure that the uterus is not filling up with blood (as described earlier)

help emergency team or flying squad to set up blood transfusion (Group O, Rh. negative or Rh. positive as required)
transfer patient to hospital when her condition has improved

## EMERGENCY CARE OF THE NEWBORN

### Mild asphyxia

At birth a baby is normally slightly blue and then rapidly becomes pink.

SIGNS AND SYMPTOMS

Dusky colour.
Good muscle tone.
Good cord pulsations.
Initial gasp, but respirations do not become established.

TREATMENT

Send for expert help.
Clean the air passages with a soft, clean handkerchief wrapped round one small finger (or by gentle suction with a soft catheter, if available).
Incline the baby's head downwards to drain liquor and blood from its respiratory tract.
Wrap in a warm blanket.
If available, give oxygen by face mask (2 litres per minute).

### Severe asphyxia

Severe asphyxia may be caused by a prolonged lack of oxygen in the uterus, or by damage to the brain. The latter is more likely to occur when the baby is born before the arrival of a midwife (BBA).

SIGNS AND SYMPTOMS

Grey or white colour.
Poor muscle tone.
Weak cord pulsations.
No respirations.

TREATMENT

Send for expert help.

Clear the air passages.

Give mouth-to-mouth ventilation taking care not to rupture the alveoli of the lungs. Place a piece of gauze over the baby's nose and mouth. The nurse then places her or his mouth over the nose and mouth of the baby and expels air about 15–20 times per minute.

Give external cardiac massage using 2 fingers to depress *gently* the lower parts of the sternum at 10 to 15 depressions per minute.

Keep baby warm.

## Hypothermia

Hypothermia may occur when the baby is born before arrival of a midwife (BBA). It describes the condition when the baby's temperature falls below 35° centigrade.

SIGNS AND SYMPTOMS

Baby feels cold to the touch, especially the head and extremities.

He or she is difficult to rouse.

He or she refuses feeds.

Red cheeks (this can be deceptive).

TREATMENT

Warm the baby slowly by dressing in layers of woollen clothing and covering head and extremities with bonnet, mittens and bootees.

Call for expert help and removal to hospital.

Put baby to the breast or, if available, give dextrose 5 per cent solution.

## CHAPTER 8

# Gynaecological Emergencies

Gynaecological emergencies can be summarised in several ways, but for simplicity they are considered here under the two broad headings of: disorders of early pregnancy; and non-pregnant disorders.

Disorders of early pregnancy will be considered up to 20 weeks' gestation for, although the time of viability is 28 weeks, a woman of over 20 weeks' gestation is likely to be admitted to hospital under the care of an obstetrician. This is because an obstetric unit has the facilities, and also the services of a paediatrician, for the care of any premature infant which might result.

## DISORDERS OF EARLY PREGNANCY

### Threatened abortion

Threatened abortion refers to bleeding from the placental site which is not severe enough to terminate the pregnancy. It usually occurs within the first 12 weeks (Fig. 69a).

#### SIGNS AND SYMPTOMS

Bright red, or brown vaginal loss.
Mild abdominal pain or backache.
The os is closed and the membranes are intact.

#### TREATMENT

The woman should be reassured and encouraged to lie down. Her pulse rate should be monitored and soiled sanitary pads saved for later estimation of her total blood loss. Her general practitioner should be informed or arrangements made for her transfer to hospital, or both.

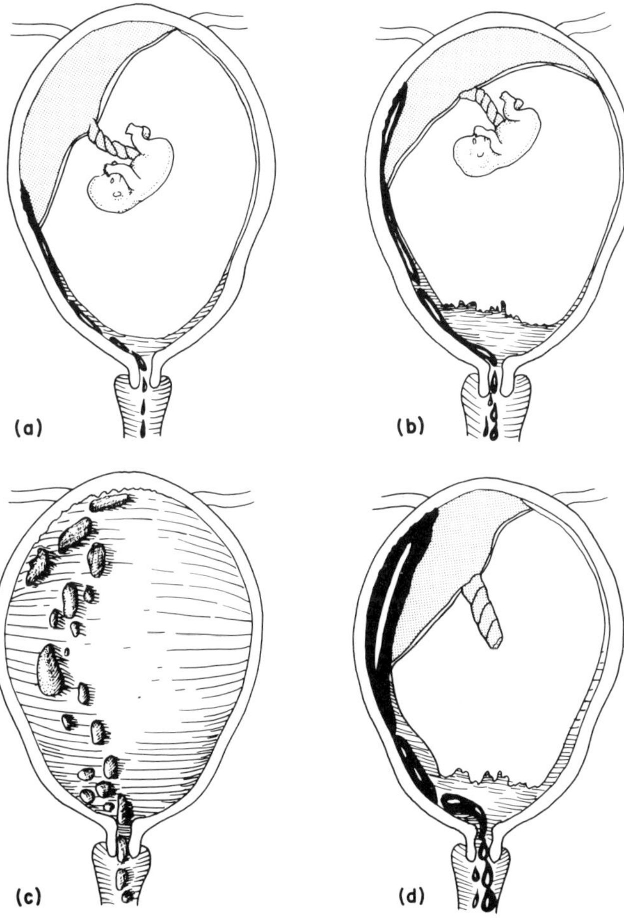


**Fig. 69** Types of abortion: (a) threatened, (b) inevitable, (c) complete and (d) incomplete.

HOSPITAL MANAGEMENT

Hospital management will consist of bed rest, sedation and tranquillisation. The patient's pulse, blood pressure and temperature will be recorded 4 hourly and her vaginal loss checked every 2 hours.

If facilities are available at the unit to which she is admitted, an ultrasound or axiscan may be performed to determine whether the fetus is still alive. It is a responsibility of the nursing staff to ensure that the patient has a full bladder for this investigation.

## Inevitable abortion

An abortion is considered to be inevitable when the cervix is dilated (Fig. 69b). This also usually occurs within the first 12 weeks of pregnancy.

### SIGNS AND SYMPTOMS

Bright red vaginal loss.
Rhythmic abdominal pain (as the uterus contracts and relaxes).
The patient is likely to be distressed, anxious and agitated.

### TREATMENT

Again the woman should be reassured and calmed as much as possible. An ambulance or her general practitioner should be summoned to take her to hospital. Before and during the journey, her pulse rate should be taken and recorded every 15 minutes and all soiled pads saved for inspection.

### HOSPITAL MANAGEMENT

Hospital management will probably consist of bedrest, and the administration of analgesics and sedatives. The patient's pulse and blood pressure will be recorded every 15 minutes to 2 hours, depending upon the severity of the bleeding. If an axiscan reveals no fetal activity or the products of conception appear through the cervix, ergometrine 0·5 mg will be ordered and given intramuscularly to encourage the uterus to expel its contents.

In *complete abortion* the whole ovum is expelled and bleeding stops fairly quickly (Fig. 69c). The patient will make a rapid physical recovery but may suffer mental stress for some time. This is more likely to be the case if the pregnancy was much wanted.

In *incomplete abortion,* the fetus is expelled but some part of the membranes or placenta are retained *in utero* (Fig. 69d). This results in the uterus being unable to contract and consequently bleeding continues. This is a fairly common outcome of an inevitable abortion.

TREATMENT

The patient should lie down and be reassured as far as possible. Arrangements for admission to hospital should be made at once. Her pulse rate and vaginal loss should be checked every 15 minutes before and during the journey and all sanitary pads saved for inspection.

HOSPITAL MANAGEMENT

Hospital treatment will include the setting up of an intravenous infusion to replace the blood volume. Observations will be continued every 15 minutes. If, on vaginal examination, the products of conception are seen in the cervical canal, they will be removed with sponge forceps. This procedure, together with an intramuscular injection of ergometrine 0·5 mg, produces a marked haemostatic effect. When her condition is satisfactory the patient will probably be taken to the theatre for curettage.

## Septic abortion

A septic abortion is one during which the patient's temperature rises. It has been seen less in Great Britain since the Abortion Act of 1967. This is because the cause is often direct interference—a criminal abortion has been attempted.

A variety of instruments or fluids may be pushed into the uterus to effect this. The most common ones are a knitting needle and soap and water injected by a Higginson's syringe. In the absence of aseptic conditions, infection occurs rapidly. The abortion goes through the stages of threatened, inevitable, and incomplete. There will be severe haemorrhage or septicaemia or both.

SIGNS AND SYMPTOMS

The important signs and symptoms are:

pallor
rapid, thready pulse
bleeding or foul-smelling bloodstained discharge *per vaginum*
abdominal pain
pyrexia
low blood pressure

TREATMENT
Treatment before admission to hospital should be the same as that described for incomplete abortion.

HOSPITAL MANAGEMENT
Hospital treatment will include intravenous infusion and antibiotics. A strict fluid balance must be kept as there is a danger of renal failure. Analgesia will also be required. Recorded observations are likely to be those relating to pulse, blood pressure, temperature and vaginal loss. These will be monitored every 15 minutes to 2 hours, depending upon the rate of bleeding. Once the infection has been brought under control, the patient will require evacuation of the uterus. This operation is necessary to stop the bleeding but must not be performed whilst there is still infection.

## Ectopic pregnancy

An ectopic pregnancy is any pregnancy which develops outside the cavity of the uterus (Plate 10). The most common site is one of the fallopian tubes, but occasionally it occurs in the abdomen or in one of the ovaries.

SIGNS AND SYMPTOMS
The signs and symptoms to look for are:
- severe abdominal pain
- tender distended abdomen
- nausea or vomiting
- rapid pulse rate
- low blood pressure
- pallor
- syncope (sometimes)
- subnormal temperature

These vary in degree according to the site of bleeding. They are most marked when there is severe intraperitoneal bleeding.

TREATMENT
It is important to get the patient to hospital as soon as possible. Whilst waiting for the ambulance, the patient should lie in the least uncomfortable position. She will be distressed and frightened and frequent verbal

reassurance will be needed. The usual observations (as previously described) should be made and recorded. Nothing should be given by mouth as an anaesthetic will be necessary on arrival at hospital.

#### HOSPITAL MANAGEMENT

Hospital treatment will be salpingectomy. Intravenous infusion will be set up as soon as possible and preparations made for taking the patient to the theatre.

In cases with slower bleeding, immediate hospital treatment may be bedrest and observation with surgery at a later stage on a routine list.

Laparoscopy is valuable in diagnosing doubtful cases.

### Hyperemesis gravidarum

Hyperemesis gravidarum is a term applied to the severe vomiting in early pregnancy, which results in metabolic changes. The patient is unable to retain solids or fluids and becomes dehydrated and ketotic.

#### TREATMENT

As it is thought that there may be a psychological reason for hyperemesis gravidarum (although it has not been proved), a sympathetic and supportive nurse can help the patient a great deal. Admission to hospital is necessary for intravenous therapy to replace fluid loss and to restore her electrolyte balance. She will also require antiemetics and tranquillisers by injection whilst the vomiting persists.

## NON-PREGNANT DISORDERS

### Acute salpingitis

Acute salpingitis may be caused by organisms reaching the fallopian tubes by ascending from the vagina (for example, gonococcus), or by direct spread from the uterus following an abortion, or from the bowel following acute appendicitis. Alternatively, the infection may be carried in the bloodstream.

#### SIGNS AND SYMPTOMS

The signs and symptoms of acute salpingitis are:

malaise

pyrexia
abdominal pain
sometimes bleeding from the vagina

TREATMENT
The patient should be encouraged to lie down until transport to hospital can be arranged. In the meantime, the usual observations relating to pulse and vaginal loss should be made and recorded. No food or fluids should be given in case a laparotomy has to be performed.

HOSPITAL MANAGEMENT
Hospital management will consist of the administration of antibiotics and analgesics. Observations will be continued; their frequency depending upon the patient's condition and blood loss. If there is any doubt about the diagnosis, a laparotomy may be necessary.

## Hydrosalpinx

The fallopian tubes may become fibrosed and thickened if an acute salpingitis is not resolved. The pus from the infection becomes a watery fluid which, unable to drain away, distends the blocked tubes. A hydrosalpinx may occur in one or both (Plate 11) of the fallopian tubes.

## Ovarian cyst

Ovarian tumours (Plate 12) are often silent and symptomless but complications which constitute emergencies can occur.

### Torsion

An ovarian cyst can twist on its pedicle when there are sudden changes in intra-abdominal pressure, such as during physical exercise. The blood supply is cut and the ovary and fallopian tube become engorged (Plate 13).

SIGNS AND SYMPTOMS
The signs and symptoms of an engorged fallopain tube are:
pallor

sweating
anxiety
rapid pulse
acute abdominal pain
nausea and vomiting
normal blood pressure

TREATMENT

The patient should be kept warm, reassured and made as comfortable as possible until admission to hospital. Nothing should be allowed by mouth as surgery will be necessary. Her pulse should be checked and recorded every 15 minutes.

HOSPITAL MANAGEMENT

Hospital management will be directed towards preparing the patient for urgent ovarian cystectomy or oophorectomy. Intravenous fluids will be initiated and the patient treated for shock.

**Rupture**

Rupture of an ovarian cyst can be either traumatic—following torsion of the pedicle; or during bimanual examination during labour when the cyst is impacted in the pelvis—or spontaneous. The latter occurs when the cyst is malignant and epithelial tissue outgrows connective tissue.

SIGNS AND SYMPTOMS

In ovarian cyst rupture, the first-aider will see the following signs and symptoms:

malaise
abdominal pain
palpable mass in the abdomen
raised pulse rate
pyrexia
nausea and vomiting
bowel sounds may or may not be present

TREATMENT

Again, operation is vital and the patient must be transported to hospital as soon as possible. She should be made as comfortable as possible and kept warm and quiet. Nothing should be given by mouth and the pulse is monitored every 15 minutes.

HOSPITAL MANAGEMENT

Hospital management may include ultrasound to confirm the diagnosis. An intravenous infusion will be set up and the patient prepared for theatre where laparotomy and cystectomy will be performed. If the cyst is malignant, the uterus, the fallopian tubes and both ovaries will be removed.

### Haemorrhage

Bleeding into the cyst may occur and will produce symptoms similar to those of torsion.

SIGNS AND SYMPTOMS

Pallor.
Anxiety.
Sweating.
Rapid pulse.
Acute abdominal pain.
Nausea and vomiting.
Low blood pressure.
Guarding and some rigidity on abdominal examination.
Palpable cyst on vaginal examination (not always).

TREATMENT

Pre-admission treatment will be similar to that described for torsion of an ovarian cyst.

HOSPITAL MANAGEMENT

Hospital management will be directed towards surgery—an ovarian cystectomy or an oophorectomy. Pre-operative care is likely to include the initiation of intravenous fluids. Until theatre is reached, observations must be made every 30 minutes.

## Carcinoma of the cervix

Carcinoma of the cervix is not generally considered as an emergency situation, but warning signs and symptoms are sometimes ignored until there is a heavy bleeding from the vagina. This can be intermenstrual; postcoital or postmenopausal or both. If the tumour is more advanced, then loss may be a heavy bloodstained, foul smelling vaginal discharge.

This is the most common tumour of the genital tract. It may have spread in the cervix or it may have formed a proliferating growth, resembling a cauliflower, protruding into the vagina (Plate 14). The latter type bleeds easily. The patient is likely to be 40 to 70 years of age.

SIGNS AND SYMPTOMS

Vaginal bleeding with no pain.
Pallor.
Sweating.
Raised pulse rate.
Low blood pressure.
Anaemia.

More commonly the patient presents with less dramatic symptoms, for example, painless vaginal bleeding with pallor. Her pulse and blood pressure may be normal.

TREATMENT

As the patient is likely to be anxious or even frightened, reassurance is important. The usual half-hourly observations should be made, until transport to hospital is available. She should be kept warm and all sanitary pads saved in order to estimate the total blood loss.

HOSPITAL MANAGEMENT

Hospital treatment will include replacement of the blood loss and routine pre-operative care, prior to a Wertheim's hysterectomy being performed. Alternatively, 4-hourly observations may be continued until a diagnostic dilation and curettage is carried out.

## Menorrhagia

Menorrhogia is heavy bleeding at the time of menstruation. The cause is likely to be fibroids, chronic inflammatory disease, endometriosis or an intra-uterine device in situ. Emotional factors should not be ruled out as contributing causes.

SIGNS AND SYMPTOMS

Heavy bleeding from the vagina.

Abdominal pain (not always).

Depending on blood loss:

pallor
rapid pulse rate
anaemia
normal to low blood pressure
normal temperature

TREATMENT

Emergency treatment will be similar to that previously described.

HOSPITAL MANAGEMENT

Hospital treatment will include replacement of the blood loss and continuation observations. When diagnosed, the underlying cause will be treated. Dilation and curettage may also be necessary to establish this.

## Dysmenorrhoea

Dysmenorrhoea is cramp-like pain at the beginning of a period. It may last for a few hours, or for a couple of days. It constitutes an emergency when it is secondary to a pelvic inflammatory disease and the pain is severe enough to cause fainting.

SIGNS AND SYMPTOMS

The signs and symptoms of dysmenorrhoea are:

acute abdominal pain
menstruation
syncope
rapid pulse rate

TREATMENT

Local warmth may provide some comfort until admission to hospital can be arranged.

HOSPITAL MANAGEMENT

Hospital management will include analgesia and the administration of antibiotics to treat the pelvic infection.

## Ovarian hyperstimulation syndrome

Ovarian hyperstimulation syndrome sometimes occurs in patients who are being treated with gonatrophins for infertility. Symptoms manifest themselves several days after administration of the hormone.

SIGNS AND SYMPTOMS

Faintness.
Lower abdominal pain.
Ascites.
Hydrothorax.

In extreme cases, there will be signs and symptoms of thrombo-embolic episodes.

TREATMENT

The patient must be admitted to hospital as quickly as possible. Emergency resuscitative procedures should be carried out as necessary.

# CHAPTER 9

# Medical Emergencies

The sudden and unexpected onset of an illness can be most alarming. It often involves the whole family, causing a fair amount of disruption and distress.

## SHOCK

Shock is difficult to define. It indicates a dynamic clinical syndrome characterised by change due to a reduction in circulatory blood volume. This causes inadequate capillary circulation leading to cellular changes.

SIGNS AND SYMPTOMS

Hypotension, tachycardia, cold clammy skin, vomiting and diminished urinary output; all leading to unconsciousness and—if not treated—death.

### Types of shock

*Mild* shock is produced by a loss of 10–20 per cent blood volume and can be easily treated.

*Severe* shock usually develops after 30 per cent blood loss. Treatment is urgent because delay will result in failure to respond adequately to transfusion, as intravascular coagulation leads to irreversible shock.

*Traumatic, oligaemic,* and *hypovolaemic* shock are terms denoting blood or plasma loss due to injury (including burns).

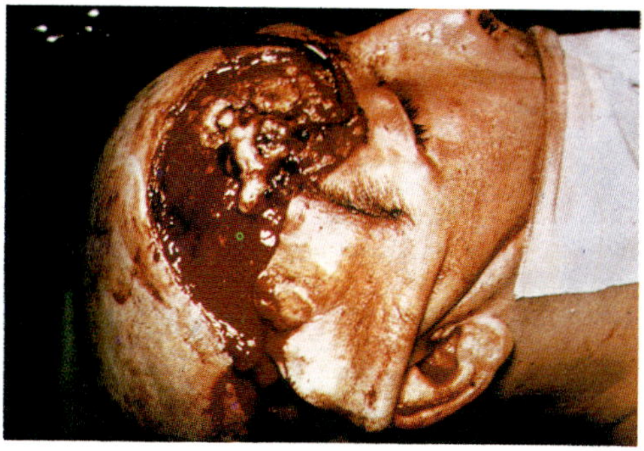

**Plate 1** Degloving of the scalp from the forehead following a road traffic accident.

**Plate 2** A deceptive serious injury of the abdomen following a pressure injury from a steering wheel. Note the slight bruising of the lower ribs and around the umbilicus. An operation revealed the complete rupture of a section of the gut.

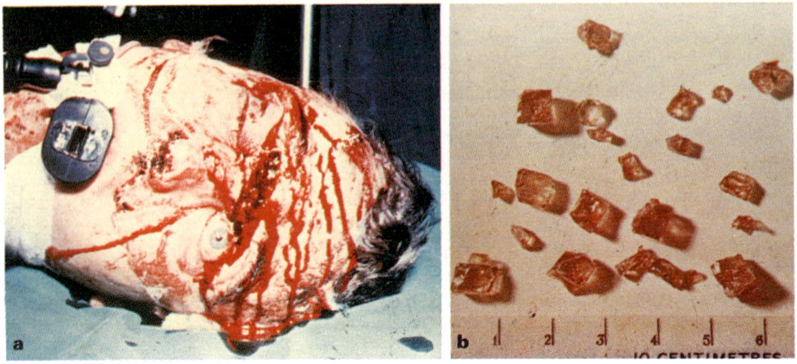


**Plate 3** Intraocular foreign bodies following a windscreen injury: (a) the left eye is swollen due to the large amount of broken glass inside and (b) the segments of glass removed from the eye. The swelling of the eye subsided after the removal of the glass.

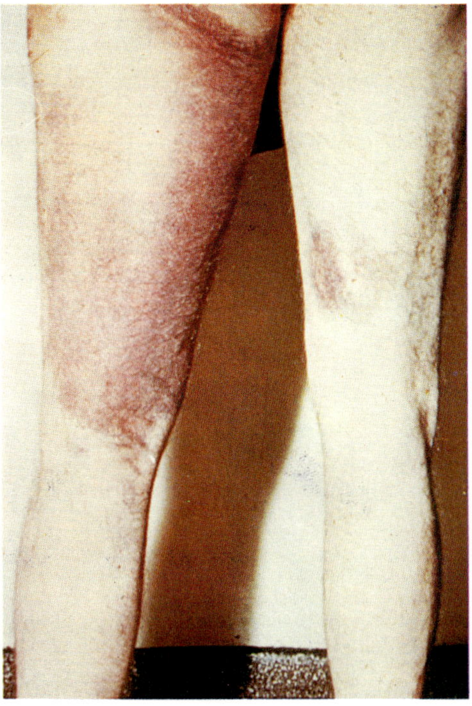

**Plate 4** Severe bruising of the thigh, representing nearly 2 litres of blood loss from the body.

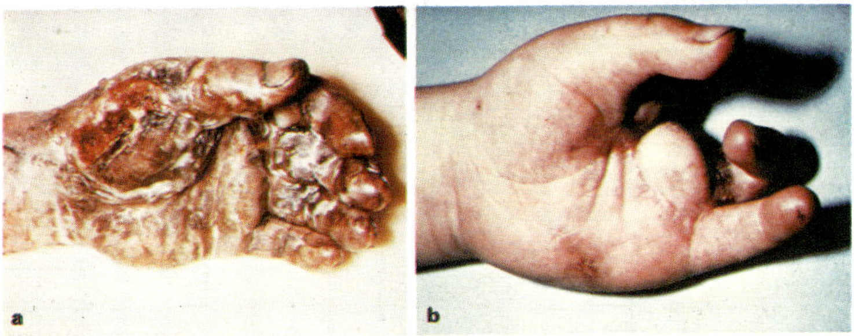

**Plate 5** A child's hand burnt by clasping the element of an electric fire showing (a) deep though non-extensive burns and (b) the resulting loss of the index and middle fingers.

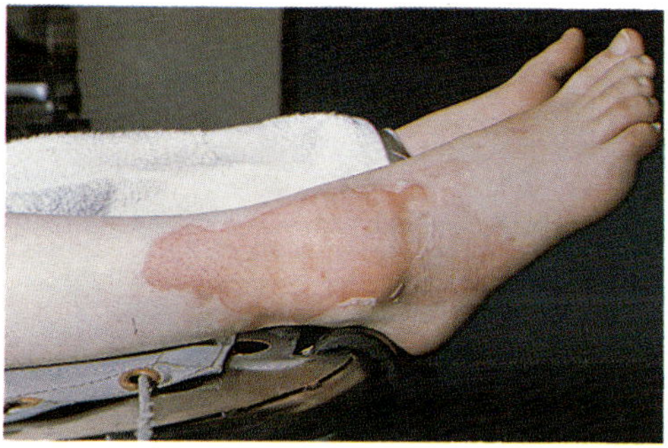

**Plate 6** Superficial burn of the ankle showing blistering and erythema.

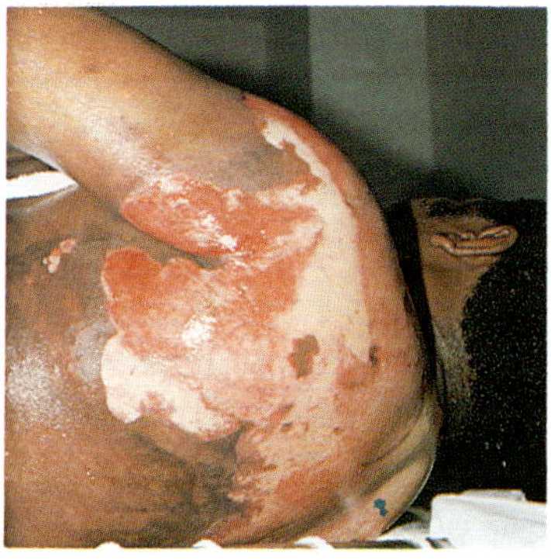

**Plate 7** Superficial and partial thickness burns: the red areas of exposed capillary bed are clearly deeper than the white areas.

**Plate 8** Very severe full thickness burn. The skin is totally destroyed exposing mainly subcutaneous tissue and even muscle fascia at the deepest point. Note the slough of charred skin on the left side and the gradual decrease in the intensity of the burn.

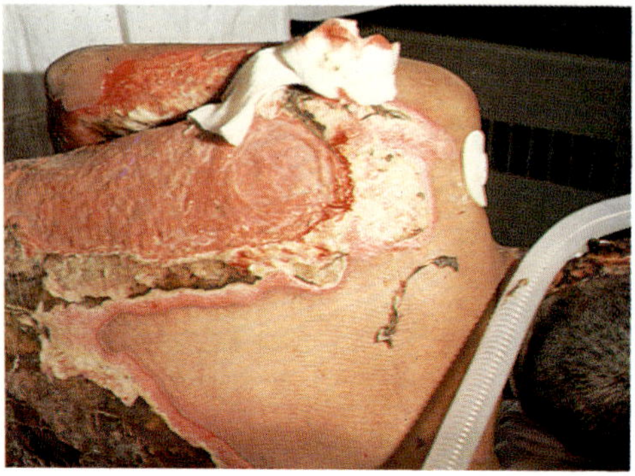

**Plate 9** Severe oedema following an extensive burn. There will be reduced circulation in the white area of skin, part of which will be completely destroyed leading to a full thickness burn. Around the edges circulation will improve.

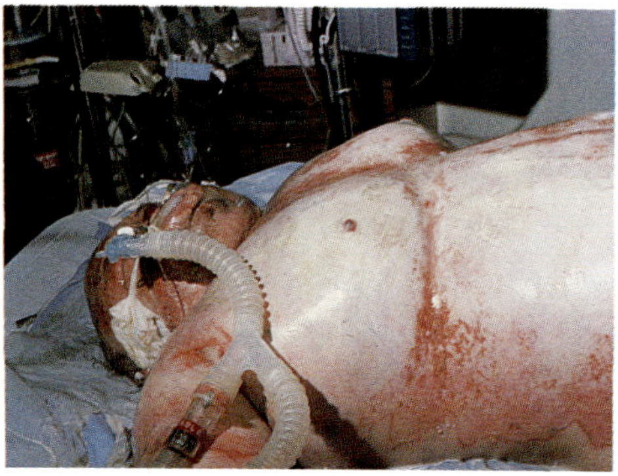

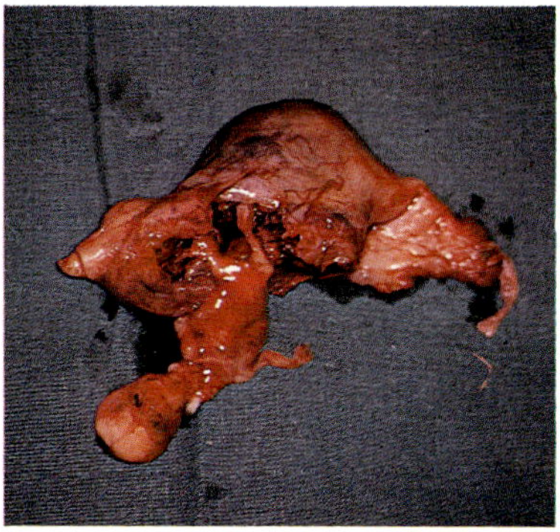

**Plate 10** An ectopic pregnancy showing the partially developed fetus.

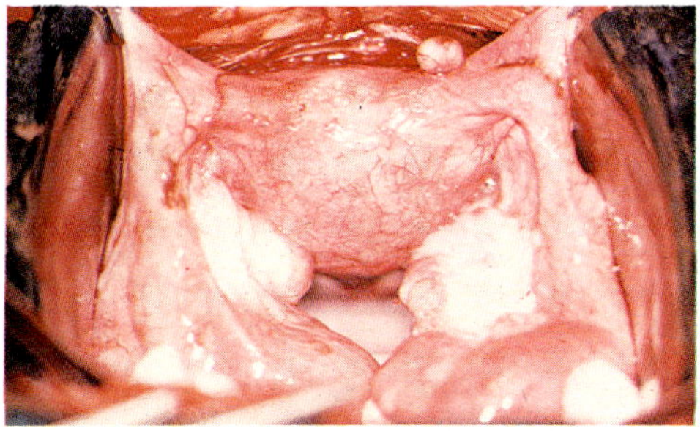

**Plate 11** A bilateral hydrosalpinx.

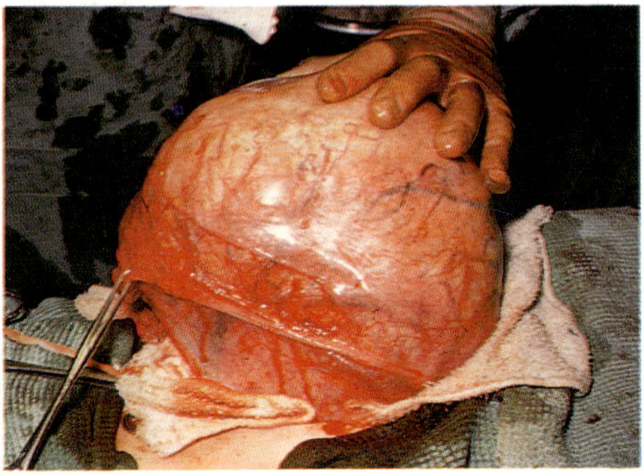

**Plate 12** Removal of a large ovarian cyst.

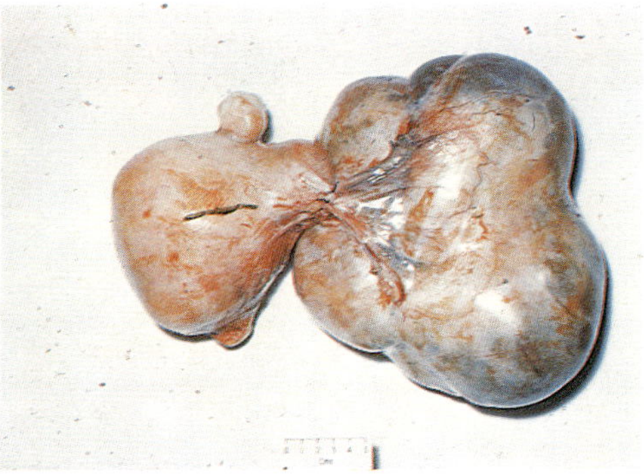

**Plate 13** An ovarian cyst twisted upon its pedicle.

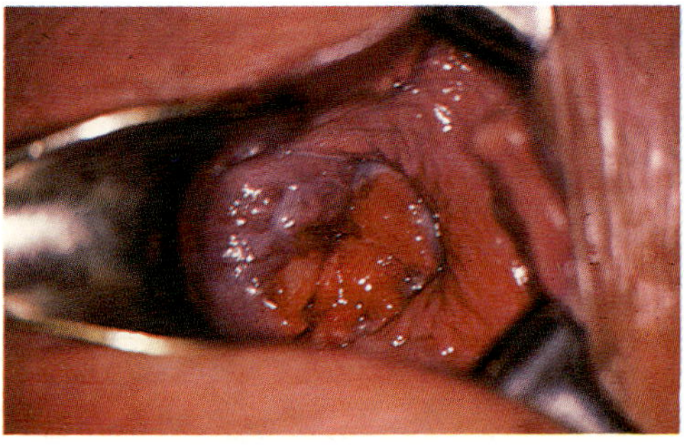

**Plate 14** Carcinoma of the cervix.

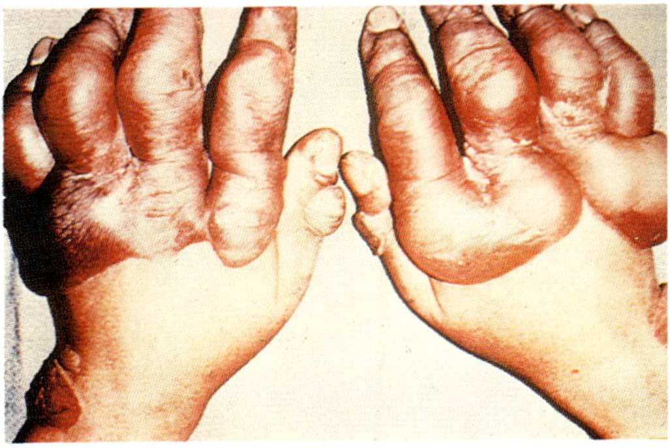

**Plate 15** A severe case of frostbite in the early stages. Note the similarity to burns.

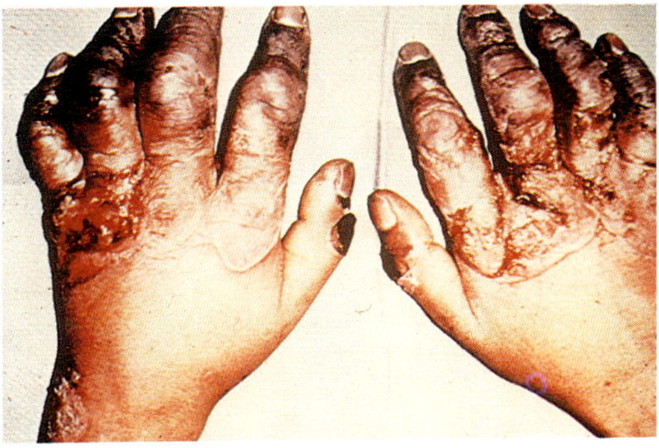

**Plate 16** The later stages of frostbite: after several days the line of demarcation is clearly visible showing areas of permanent damage at the tips of the fingers and healing areas at the bases. The gangrenous digits will require amputation.

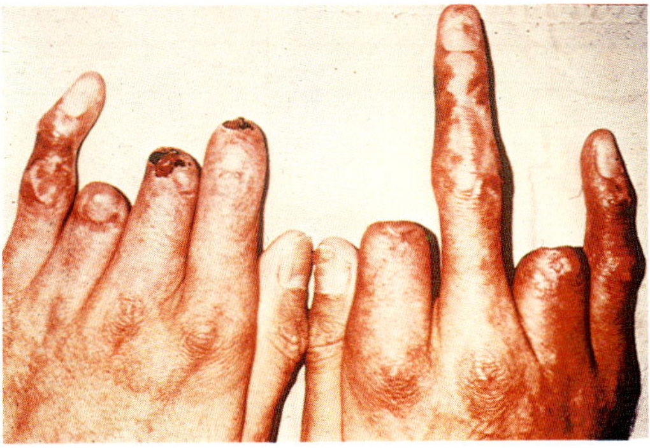

**Plate 17** Amputations have been carried out through the joints as a result of the frostbite. Note the slowness of the skin to heal over the tips of the stumps and the scarring of the remaining fingers.

*Cardiac* shock is due to heart failure.

*Toxic* shock is the result of sepsis.

*Neurogenic* shock is a psychological phenomenon often brought about by emotion or by experiencing pain.

*Spinal* shock follows damage to the spinal cord at the cervical or upper thoracic level.

*Anaphylactic* shock is an extreme form of hypersensitivity on injection of a foreign protein. Adrenaline may restore normal vascular tone.

*Endocrine* shock is a crisis condition seen in certain diseases such as Addison's disease. Again there is hypotension, hypothermia and sometimes unconsciousness.

## CARDIAC ISCHAEMIA

Probably the most dramatic sudden illness is that due to cardiac ischaemia. The heart is a muscle and all muscles need an adequate blood supply at all times. The cutting off of the blood supply, either by spasm or a blockage in the vessels, results in ischaemia. Spasm of the coronary vessels supplying the heart muscle is known as angina, whilst coronary thrombosis is a blockage of the artery.

Ischaemic hypoxia occurs when there is obstruction of an artery (for example, the basilar artery). Capillaries are rendered more permeable than normal and this causes plasma to pass into the tissues where acid metabolites form.

### SIGNS AND SYMPTOMS

In either case, the patient experiences frightening and severe pain in the chest; the pain radiates down the arms and up the neck into the jaw. 'Seized with pain' is a very good description, as the victim is unable to move and often clutches at his or her chest. In severe cases, the heart stops beating and death is instantaneous. Cardiac resuscitation and artificial respiration should always be attempted, however, as prompt action may save life.

### TREATMENT

In less severe cases, when the patient does not lose consciousness, no attempt should be made to move him or her; a chair should be brought so that he or she can sit down. The patient's own doctor should be called. If the doctor is able to come straight away, the patient should be left where he or she is. If, however, there is going to be a delay before the doctor can visit, the patient may be moved to a comfortable armchair, settee or bed, whichever is conveniently available. If possible, the move should be made by carrying the patient on the chair on which he or she is already sitting. If there is no one available to lift, the patient may walk, slowly and with assistance, when he or she feels able to do so. It is helpful to keep a record of the pulse rate, taken at 15 minute intervals. These patients often feel sick, and may vomit, so the first-aider should have a bowl and tissues in readiness should this occur. The patient should be kept quiet and undisturbed until the doctor arrives. Relatives will need reassurance also, and if they are obviously frightened, it is better to keep them away from the room in which the patient is resting.

## LOSS OF CONSCIOUSNESS

Loss of consciousness is another medical emergency which is frightening to the relatives. There are many causes for this condition. Some of the commoner causes of unconsciousness are:

- syncope or fainting
- cerebrovascular accident or stroke
- coma from diabetes mellitus

#### TREATMENT

In every case the basic principles of first aid treatment are to:

- ensure that there is a clear airway
- institute artificial respiration and cardiac resuscitation if breathing and heart stop
- prevent further injury
- obtain medical help as soon as possible

### Syncope or fainting

Fainting occurs when the brain has insufficient blood for its needs. This occurs in someone who has been standing for a long time, especially in hot, overcrowded conditions. It may also accompany diarrhoea and vomiting in food poisoning, or may be induced by the sight of something upsetting, for example, a road traffic accident. The victim is pale, often perspiring, and falls to the ground as consciousness is lost.

TREATMENT

Once the casualty is in a horizontal position, the blood supply to the brain improves and consciousness returns. The patient should therefore be kept flat and should not attempt to sit up until he or she has fully recovered. People who faint in crowded conditions are in some danger, unless the crowd can be moved back from them. If this is not possible, the casualty should be carried, preferably on a stretcher if one is available, to an area where there is some space and fresh air. As the patient recovers, colour will return and he or she will probably feel better quite quickly. A drink of water or tea, if available, is usually appreciated.

People sometimes feel faint without actually losing consciousness. In such cases, the casualty's head should be lowered, either by putting it between the knees, or by laying the person flat on the floor. Recovery is usually rapid.

In the majority of cases, people recover from a faint quickly and no further treatment is necessary. If, however, fainting is persistent and the patient continues to feel ill, medical advice should be sought.

## Cerebrovascular accident or stroke

All body movement and functions are controlled by the brain, which is an exceedingly complex organ. But, like all other organs, the brain is dependent on a steady and sufficient blood supply. Any alteration in the blood supply to the brain will show itself by a loss of function or movement of some part of the body and such an attack is known as a stroke.

Strokes vary in extent and severity according to the size of the brain area involved. They range from transient losses of consciousness, followed by numbness or tingling of a set of muscles, to such severe damage that the patient never regains consciousness before death. In many cases, the patient loses consciousness for a period of time, then regains it with paralysis of one side of the body and sometimes affections of speech. As far as first aid is concerned, the situation is one in which someone has become unconscious.

The victim is usually elderly and there may be a history of raised blood pressure. The patient may have complained of feeling unwell prior to the emergency, but equally may have appeared in good health and spirits. The circumstances are similarly varied; the loss of consciousness may occur whilst the person is in an armchair or in bed; he or she may be walking in the street, playing golf or bowls, or driving a car. The situation may therefore be a straightforward one or it may be much more complicated. Someone who has a stroke whilst driving a car, for instance, may not be the only victim of a road traffic accident involving several people. Someone who has a stroke at the top of a flight of stairs may fall down the flight and be found unconscious at the bottom. Each case must therefore be considered on its own merits, but the first-aider must invariably deal with the unconscious casualty.

TREATMENT

As in every case of unconsciousness, it is essential to check that the patient is breathing. If not, artificial respiration must be started, and, if necessary, cardiac resuscitation also.

Further help will be needed. If the stroke has occurred out of doors, a passer-by or someone in a nearby house should be asked to telephone for an ambulance. Whilst awaiting its arrival the patient should be arranged in a position which ensures a clear airway. If lying in a position of danger, for example, in the street, the patient could be lifted to the pavement; otherwise it is better to leave him or her until the ambulance arrives. Only if the weather is very bad, or the ambulance long delayed should the patient be carried to a place of shelter.

If the stroke has occurred in the patient's home, the doctor should be notified immediately. Whilst awaiting his or her arrival, the patient should be arranged in a position which ensures a clear airway, and kept quiet.

The relatives should be comforted; asking them to do something such as making a pot of tea will help. The doctor will either keep the patient in bed at home, or transfer him or her to hospital, so the relatives can also make preparations for either eventuality.

Should the patient recover consciousness before the doctor arrives, he or she should not be moved, but kept quiet and reassured.

## Diabetes mellitus

The onset of diabetes is usually a gradual process.

### SIGNS AND SYMPTOMS

The person feels thirsty and drinks more, so passes more urine; he or she loses weight and does not feel at all well. If these symptoms are disregarded, the patient can lapse into coma. If diabetes has not been diagnosed, there will be no indication as to why the patient is unconscious. He or she will be in urgent need of treatment in hospital, and should be transferred there as soon as possible.

### TREATMENT

Once diabetes has been diagnosed, treatment is instituted and the object of this is to achieve a balance between the food the patient eats and the amount of insulin required to metabolise the food. This process of stabilisation often has to be done in hospital and sometimes proves a difficult process. Once achieved, however, the person can live a normal life with the diabetes controlled, but not cured. Control has to be exercised at all times and the danger is that events may upset this fine balance.

If diabetic patients have too much carbohydrate and fat in their diet without an adequate amount of insulin, they will become comatose; similarly, if they have too much insulin and insufficient food, they will also go into a coma. When diabetic patients are stabilised at the start of their illness, they are taught how to recognise the first symptoms of coma and what to do when or if they appear. Sometimes, however, a diabetic patient fails to take appropriate action, and the first-aider may have to deal with the result. If a known diabetic feels faint, begins to sweat, looks ill, and is confused, he or she should be given sugar at once. The sugar may be in the form of a sugar lump, a spoonful of honey, or a sweet drink. If the symptoms are due to too much insulin, the administration of sugar will relieve the symptoms immediately and the patient will recover. If the opposite is the cause of the developing coma, the small amount of sugar will not make any material difference. The patient must be transferred to hospital without delay.

Many diabetic patients carry some form of identification with them, for example, a 'medic alert' bracelet or card in their pocket or handbag. It is always worthwhile to look for these.

When ketonuria is the only clinical evidence of ketosis, treatment depends upon whether the patient is on insulin, and if so, its type and dosage.

The blood sugar level at which symptoms and signs of hypoglycaemia appear varies in different patients, but is typically not higher than *50 mg per 100 ml* unless the rate of the fall is very rapid.

Hypoglycaemic and diabetic coma are not alike but for those who seldom see unconscious diabetics, the main differential features are summarised in Table 1.

**Table 1** Difference between hypoglycaemic and diabetic coma

| | Hypoglycaemic coma | Diabetic coma |
|---|---|---|
| Mode of onset | Sudden | Gradual |
| Respiration | As in sleep | Deep abdominal (air hunger) |
| Acetone in breath | Absent | Present |
| Tongue | Moist | Dry and furred |
| Skin | Moist | Dry |
| Blood pressure | Normal | Low |
| Ocular tension | Normal | Low |
| Ketonuria | Absent or slight | Heavy |
| Glycosuria | Variable | Heavy |
| Blood sugar | Less than 60 mg per cent | More than 300 mg per cent |

## EPILEPSY

An epileptic fit is a frightening experience for all concerned.

### SIGNS AND SYMPTOMS

The person may give a loud cry before falling unconscious to the ground. He or she will lose control of the muscles which will contract violently; he or she may be incontinent of urine and foam at the mouth. If the patient bites his or her tongue during the attack, this foam will be bloodstained.

### TREATMENT

The aim of the first-aid treatment is to prevent the patient from injuring himself or herself during an attack. Fortunately the period of time is short and the patient usually recovers fairly quickly. He or she should be kept quiet until fully recovered and then be escorted home.

Once an epileptic fit has occurred, the patient should consult a general practitioner. The condition can be controlled by drugs and further fits will be unlikely.

## ACUTE ABDOMINAL EMERGENCIES

There are a large number of conditions which cause acute abdominal pain. A person can deteriorate considerably because no one recognises that the situation is urgent and, therefore, delay summoning a doctor. First-aiders should therefore be alert to recognise those signs and symptoms which require urgent attention, because they herald serious illness.

#### SIGNS AND SYMPTOMS

Persistent pain should never be ignored. When the person is in such severe pain that he or she is unable to move, or rolls about in agony, it is obvious that a doctor should be summoned. But someone in rather less pain may attempt to make light of it. In such cases, the pulse rate is a valuable guide. A raised pulse rate is a danger sign, and if the rate goes on rising, then the condition is a serious one. A pale, sweating person who is restless, has a raised pulse rate, dry furred tongue and abdominal pain, should be seen by a doctor without delay.

#### TREATMENT

Whilst awaiting the doctor's arrival, nothing should be given by mouth; any vomit should be saved and if the patient passes urine or faeces, these should also be saved for inspection. The patient should be kept quiet and reassured. A written record should be kept of the pulse rate and the times at which he or she was sick, or complained of a different type of pain.

### Food poisoning

Acute abdominal pain often accompanies an attack of food poisoning and this condition can be alarming. The person suddenly feels ill and experiences pain, diarrhoea and sickness, often simultaneously. In mild cases, the condition clears up fairly quickly once the poisonous food has been eliminated. The patient will fetl weak and tired, however, and should rest.

Persistent vomiting and diarrhoea is another matter, as people can quickly become dehydrated, especially if they are very young or very old. In such cases a doctor should be summoned. Any food thought to be the cause of the attack should be saved for examination. In the event of a number of people suffering from the signs and symptoms of food poisoning, investigations will be made to try to establish the cause of the outbreak. Both doctors and public health inspectors will be involved in the investigation; the first-aider should save and label any specimens and hand them over when asked to do so.

## POISONING AND TOXIC REACTIONS

In addition to poisoning by food and the swallowing of poisons as such (see pages 161–4), people sometimes do produce reactions to drugs, and these must also be recognised. Some drugs, especially antibiotics, can cause a rash and the sudden appearance of a rash on someone who is taking drugs should be regarded as a danger signal. The patient's doctor should be notified. The doctor will decide whether it is in the patient's best interest to stop the drug or not. Other drugs can cause indigestion and vomiting. In these cases, it is wise to withhold further doses of the drug until the doctor has been consulted.

Some medicines have specific reactions and the patient or relatives will have been warned about them. Even so, they do not always recognise them when they arise. Digitalis, e.g., a useful drug in many heart conditions, accumulates after a time in the body and signs and symptoms of overdose appear. The patient will not seem well and lose his or her appetite, especially for sweet foods. If the pulse rate is below normal and the beats are coupled, the patient almost certainly has accumulated too much digitalis. The doctor must be notified and in the meantime, no further doses should be given.

Many modern drugs are complex substances and a reaction to them may occur if taken with certain foods. Patients are told of these dangers, but, again, they sometimes disregard or forget the advice they have been given. If a person who is taking medicine for some condition suddenly feels very ill, has a raised pulse rate or is sick, careful enquiry should be made about what he or she has had to eat and drink. It may well be that the symptoms are due to a reaction between the drug and the food.

### Alcohol

Alcohol is especially prone to react with drugs and the person may well be thought to be hopelessly drunk. This reaction may have developed after only one small drink, however, and this fact should lead to making the correct diagnosis. The patient should be kept quiet in bed and the doctor notified.

### Allergy

Allergic reactions to drugs or food or even something the person inhales can also occur. Allergy is a specific reaction of the body to foreign protein and it shows itself in a number of ways. There may be severe running of the eyes and nose, or there may be difficulty in breathing. A rash may appear on the skin, or there may be swelling of the mucous membrane, especially of the throat and mouth. The person is usually frightened, unless he or she has had previous attacks and knows what is happening. The patient should be reassured and medical attention should be sought without delay. If the person has already been treated for allergy, he or she may already have a remedy. This should be given immediately.

## HEAT RELATED EMERGENCIES

Under normal circumstances, the human body is capable of maintaining its own internal temperature at a constant level of 36–37° C. The physiological mechanisms responsible are complex ones but amazingly efficient; whether the weather or environment is hot or cold, the body temperature remains constant. There are very few conditions which upset this equilibrium, so extremes of body temperature are comparatively uncommon.

### Hypothermia

A fall in the body temperature is a condition which may arise in the very young or the very old (Fig. 70).

**In the very young**
The heat-regulating centre in babies needs a few weeks to adjust from

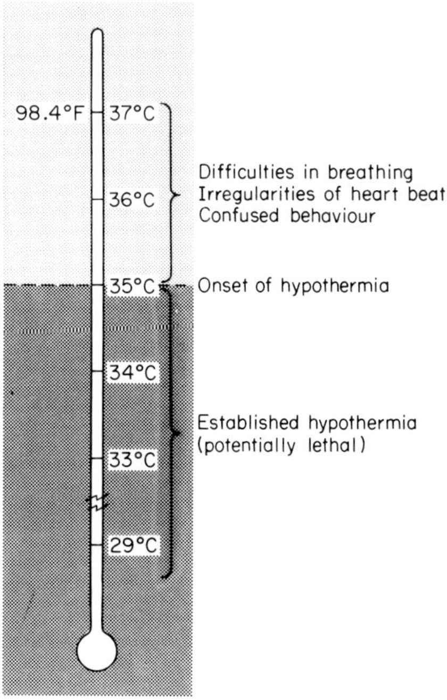


**Fig. 70** A fall in body temperature and its effects.

the environment of the womb to that of the world. An infant also has a larger surface area in relation to its body weight, so heat loss is relatively great (Fig. 71). The temperature of the nursery should not be allowed to fall too low, and wide fluctuations in temperature must be avoided. Whilst babies need fresh air like everyone else, they must not be left in cold bedrooms with a window wide open. If it is impossible to warm the room the baby should have a hot water bottle—well wrapped up and placed under the mattress.

SIGNS AND SYMPTOMS

A baby suffering from hypothermia will be pale and lethargic; it will be difficult to get him or her to suck. The skin will be cold to touch and if a low reading thermometer is available, a temperature below normal will be registered.

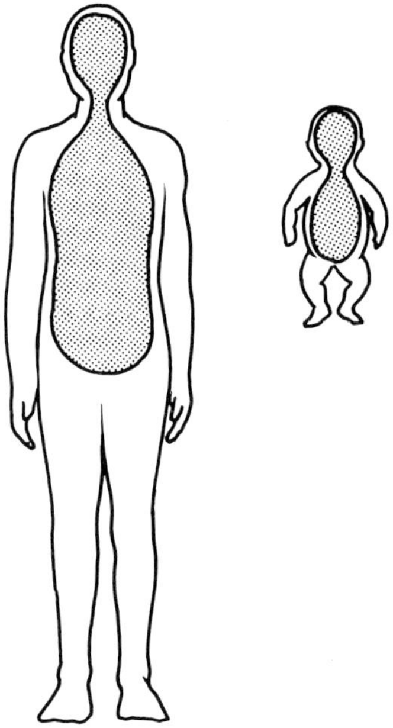

**Fig. 71** Temperature cores showing an infant's relatively larger surface area for a small body mass.

TREATMENT

Treatment consists of warming the baby. This can be done by wrapping the baby in a blanket and keeping him or her in a warm atmosphere. If no heat is available, the baby should be held, carefully wrapped in an eiderdown or duvet. Medical advice should be sought without delay.

**In the very old**

The very old tend to lose their ability to adapt to cold conditions. Because they are old and frail, they move slowly and take little exercise; therefore less body heat is generated. Old people who live alone frequently find that cooking meals is a chore which becomes too much of a burden. They tend to eat foods which do not contain all the essential items of nutrition, for example, tea and buns or biscuits, because these are easy to prepare. The high cost of any form of heating means that elderly people with a small income cannot afford to heat their homes adequately. The cumulative effect of all these factors may produce a state of hypothermia and this condition is not an uncommon one amongst old people during a cold winter.

The condition is also seen in elderly people who are unexpectedly exposed to cold for a long period. Someone who gets up at night to go to the lavatory, falls and breaks a leg and lies for several hours clad only in a nightdress or pyjamas in a cold house, may also suffer from hypothermia.

#### SIGNS AND SYMPTOMS

Hypothermia should be suspected if an elderly person is found in an apathetic and confused state in a very cold room. The face will be pale and the skin cold to touch. District nurses and health visitors who are on the alert for this condition, are often equipped with special low reading thermometers, and the use of one of these will confirm the diagnosis. If the temperature is below 28° C the pulse must be carefully monitored as ventricular fibrillation can occur.

#### TREATMENT

Treatment consists of warming both the patient and the environment by whatever means available. A fire or stove should be lit, open windows closed and the patient wrapped in an eiderdown, duvet or blankets. A well-covered hot water bottle can be used to warm the surrounding blanket or covers. A hot, sweet drink may be given. A message should be sent to the patient's own general practitioner. These patients should not be warmed rapidly at the outset as a sudden change in temperature can lead to circulatory collapse.

If the patient is found in conditions where heat cannot be supplied, such as a flat or house bereft of gas or electricity or means of lighting a fire, an ambulance should be called to transport the patient to hospital.

## Exposure

### Hypothermia

Hypothermia can also occur in young people if they are exposed to wet, cold conditions and fail to take proper precautions. People who venture out in mountainous or fell country with inadequate footwear and clothing are at risk if a storm breaks or a thick mist suddenly descends; the risk is obviously greater if they are lost or injured. In such a case, there is fairly rapid mental and physical deterioration, followed by loss of consciousness; death will follow unless the person is rescued.

Rescue is usually undertaken by a prepared and equipped team, who are trained and have had experience in similar difficult conditions.

TREATMENT

The aim of treatment is to shelter the person from further exposure by covering the person with a tent or plastic bag or sleeping bag and then to carry him or her to a place of safety where further resuscitative measures can be instituted.

If possible, at that point, the patient should be placed in a bath of water kept at a constant temperature of 42–44° C. After about 10 minutes, there should be signs of recovery; the patient should then be transferred to bed in a warm room. When possible a doctor should be present during the re-warming procedure.

**Effect of lightning**

Lightning may produce bizarre effects, frequently stripping clothing to shreds. Patches of scorching may occur on the skin and lacerated wounds if metallic objects are in contact. Shock will be severe and resuscitation may be necessary.

## Frostbite

Frostbite is rarely seen in the United Kingdom, as it only occurs when the temperature falls below −1° C, but cases can occur in severe winters.

The areas most likely to be frostbitten are fingers, toes, cheeks, nose and ears (see also page 81).

SIGNS AND SYMPTOMS

The danger signs are intense coldness of the part, followed by a loss of sensation. When pressed, the tissues will feel soft.

TREATMENT

If the part can be warmed at this stage, recovery is rapid. The affected area should be covered up, preferably with something warm, such as a scarf or mittens and the casualty wrapped in a rug. As soon as possible, the patient should go into a house or building where the temperature is warm or at least above freezing point.

### Deep frostbite

In a situation where warming cannot take place and the person remains exposed to severe cold, deep frostbite may occur (Plate 15). In this condition, there is a loss of sensation, the area feels very cold to touch and the tissues, when pressed, are hard and unyielding. This condition requires expert medical attention and the casualty must be transported to it as quickly as possible. Re-warming must take place where there are proper facilities for aftercare, as once the area has been warmed it must not be allowed to freeze again. This is why first aid treatment should not be attempted under the cold conditions. If frostbite is not treated with urgency, the extremities will become gangrenous and require amputation (Plates 16 and 17).

## Heatstroke

The United Kingdom lies in a temperate zone, it is very rare for air temperatures to reach such heights that people suffer from heatstroke.

### In children

Small children who are exposed to the summer sun on the beach where there is no shade do sometimes show signs of overheating.

#### SIGNS AND SYMPTOMS

The child so affected will appear very flushed and the skin feels excessively hot and dry. The tongue will be dry and the child fretful and unhappy.

#### TREATMENT

Treatment consists of putting the child in a shady place with a free current of air, and sponging the skin with tepid water. The skin should not be dried: the water should be allowed to evaporate. Plenty of drinks must be given. As soon as practicable the child should be transported home and kept quiet in a cool, shaded room until seen by a doctor.

### In adults

Adults rarely suffer from heatstroke due to climatic conditions in the United Kingdom, but sometimes the skin gets burnt when people stay in direct sunlight for some hours. If a breeze is blowing, they do not feel too hot, but the action of the sun's rays on the skin may cause redness and blistering. This condition is especially likely to occur in young people at the start of a summer holiday. They sunbathe with great enthusiasm without adequately protecting the skin first.

TREATMENT

Treatment is to cover the burnt area with clothing and get the casualty home or back to the hotel. Then the area can be sponged with cool water or saline. Any blisters should be left alone. A dressing may be necessary in severe cases and a dose of a mild analgesic will relieve the discomfort and pain. Further sunbathing should be forbidden until the skin has healed and even then, the person should be very careful; this advice is usually accepted without demur.

### Heat exhaustion

In certain manufacturing processes, notably mining and steel and iron casting, workers may be exposed to very high temperatures. Proper precautions are taken to avoid the onset of heat exhaustion in these conditions and the workers are trained to be on the alert for early signs and symptoms.

SIGNS AND SYMPTOMS

The affected person loses both fluid and salt through the skin; he or she is hot and dehydrated, and feels ill. The loss of salt causes muscular cramp which may be severe.

TREATMENT

Treatment consists of removing the casualty at once from the hot atmosphere and giving saline to drink. Salt tablets are kept in the first aid kit of mines and factories for this purpose. The casualty should rest in the first aid room before being allowed to go home.

## ANIMAL BITES/SCRATCHES

To be bitten by a dog is a frightening experience as well as a painful one. Fortunately most bites are superficial and although there may be profuse bleeding, the wound is not usually serious. The laceration should be washed, preferably under running water, and a dry dressing applied. It is wise to advise the casualty to see his or her own doctor, as protection against tetanus may be required. Any continued pain, swelling and redness of the wound will indicate the onset of sepsis, and a doctor should then be consulted without delay.

Cats do not bite, but they do scratch and sometimes they attack children and even adults—another very frightening experience. Once a cat's claws have embedded themselves in the skin, the cat will not let go. Pulling it only makes the wounds deeper and longer, so the cat must be hit on the head, unkind though this may seem. The scratches bleed profusely. The wounds should be washed, preferably under running water, and dry dressings applied. The casualty should be advised to consult a doctor as these scratches may well be infected from the cat's claws.

## INSECT STINGS

Bees and wasps are the two insects in this country which sting humans. The bee leaves its sting in the tissues, but the wasp does not. A wasp can therefore sting a person more than once.

Bee stings should be removed from the skin as soon as possible. They can usually be seen and can be pulled out with forceps, eyebrow tweezers, or sometimes even a finger and thumb. The part feels sore and there is local swelling; a solution of sodium bicarbonate swabbed on to the area gives relief. Occasionally, the toxin in the sting gives rise to a severe general reaction, known as anaphylactic shock. The casualty looks ill and pale, sweats, and may develop a generalised urticarial rash. Coma and death may follow in severe cases. This condition requires medical attention urgently, and the casualty must go to hospital or be seen by a doctor, whichever is the quicker.

Severe reaction also follows numerous stings; again medical attention must be obtained without delay.

The pain of a wasp sting can be relieved by swabbing the part with an acid solution such as vinegar or lemon juice. Generalised reactions do not occur so frequently as with bee stings, but someone who is attacked by a swarm of wasps will be very ill and must have immediate medical attention.

# CHAPTER 10

# Poisoning

Poison is a substance that when absorbed by a living organism kills or injures it. It may be absorbed by ingestion, by inhalation, intravenously, through the skin or by any other route. The effect may be instantaneous, quick, slow, or cumulative.

At present there are approximately 120 000 hospital admissions for acute poisoning annually in England and Wales. In 1978 the combined National Poisons Information Services handled about 40 000 telephone enquiries. The service they provide is intended primarily as an Information Service for staff dealing with acute emergencies (see Appendix 2).

Laws have been passed and regulations formulated to protect people from poisoning by drugs, and nurses should keep themselves informed about such legislation and support all measures aimed to provide public protection. In hospitals, drugs of a highly poisonous potential are kept locked up. Some toxic antiseptic solutions are often to be seen in treatment and operating rooms, however, and these also can cause death. As it is difficult always to recognise potential suicides, all lotions and medicines should be made as inaccessible as possible to patients.

While poisoning by contaminated food and by therapeutic drugs is occurring more frequently, ingestion of poison by mistake or by intent is also a fairly common emergency. (Drug addiction with consequent illnesses and deaths is a subject on its own and discussion of it as a social problem is not appropriate in a practical textbook of this nature.) Much more can be done to prevent the swallowing of poison by mistake.

## HOUSEHOLD POISONS

All medicines, bleaches, and disinfectants should be kept well out of reach of children and mentally ill, confused, deficient or retarded people.

Particularly dangerous household fluids are:

| | |
|---|---|
| ammonia | oven cleaners |
| antifreeze liquid | paintbrush restorers |
| bleaches | paint stripper |
| caustic soda | pest poisons |

Fluids should never be transferred from one bottle to another. It is easy to forget that a lemonade bottle has been used for strong bleaching fluid, and other people will not be aware of it.

Pesticides, in addition to being toxic, may be inflammable; their use and storage should be carefully supervised. They should not be stored, for example, in an area used for cooking or serving food.

### TREATMENT

The treatment of a poisoned individual should be given as a matter of extreme urgency; this is one of those emergencies where time is of the essence. As some authorities point out, time should not be spent in trying to find causes and antidotes before beginning treatment. Such minutes could well cost the patient's life. The patient should be taken to hospital at once.

The three steps advocated by the majority of experts are:

remove the poison from the body
administer antidotes
give symptomatic and supportive treatment

Poison is usually removed from the stomach most effectively by gastric lavage, but this can be contraindicated when the poison is highly corrosive or is a convulsive drug (for example, strychnine). In the former case the gastric tube could perforate the already injured oesophagus or stomach, and in the latter instance, the procedure could stimulate further fits. Sometimes a saline cathartic is introduced by the lavage-tube after the stomach is washed out.

Emetics are advocated by some people but the current thinking is that they are of value 'only in rare cases'. Sometimes they can be a greater danger: instances where salt and water in strong proportions have been given, for example, have led to death. Apomorphine given hypodermically is the most rapidly effective emetic. Mustard water in the proportion of one teaspoonful to a glass of tepid water is sometimes used when gastric lavage and apomorphine are not available. Needless to say, vomiting should not be induced in unconscious patients.

### In the young

Children sometimes present a problem when the stomach contents are tablets that are too large to be drawn through the small size tube. The most effective way to induce vomiting in an 'under 5 year old' is to give a large dose of ipecac (15 ml followed by another 10–15 ml if vomiting does not occur within 15 minutes). In the USA some physicians prescribe a 1 oz dose of ipecac for all children so that parents may have it always at hand. In Britain we advise parents to take their children to hospital or a doctor straight away. As a small island, few people are far from medical help of one kind or another. Strong salt solutions should **never** be used. Vomiting should not be induced in children who have swallowed caustics as this would mean that the oesophagus would be injured once more.

Lead poisoning is a serious environmental hazard for young children and one which is theoretically preventable. Cots, playpens, and the like should not be covered with lead-containing paint and small children should be carefully supervised if lead pipes and paint become accessible to them in other situations.

### Antidotes

Antidotes for some poisons are known and the Poisons Centres within the United Kingdom will always give emergency advice (see Appendix 2). Antidotes are of two kinds: chemical and physiological. Chemical antidotes inactivate the poison by chemical reaction, whilst physiological antidotes combat the harmful physiological effect of the poison. For an alkali poisoning, an acid such as vinegar is a chemical antidote, while a physiological antidote for a poison which has caused respiratory depression would be a drug which stimulates respiration. Frank poisons usually give the antidote on the label, but cleaning fluids, insect and animal poisons and the like rarely do. Antidotes as a water solution are sometimes effectively used in gastric lavage.

Even when the antidote is known, it is seldom immediately available. The following are some of the few which are usually found in every household:

For poisoning by a heavy metal  Milk and egg white.

For poisoning by an irritant such as iodine  Flour and starch water.

For poisoning by an alkaloid  Strong tea and diluted tincture of iodine.

Unless one is far away from medical help, time should not be wasted in hunting for any antidote; the best move is to send for medical aid or get the victim to a hospital.

Many ingested poisons are eliminated by the kidneys and patients should therefore be encouraged to drink as much water as possible. This will dilute the toxic substance and so minimise harmful effects on the kidneys.

The elimination of volatile substances by the lungs can sometimes be speeded by stimulating respiration.

If the poison has not been swallowed but is in contact with the skin, repeated bathing in running water is the most effective treatment. If the irritant is insoluble in water a bland substance that will dissolve the toxic substance, such as vegetable oil or alcohol according to the nature of the poison, should be used.

When contact with a poisonous plant is suspected, scrubbing with yellow laundry soap is sometimes effective. (Some susceptible people are 'immunised' to prevent such an occurrence, but this is not always one-hundred per cent proof, especially in controlling the effects of poisonous ivy and the like).

## GAS POISONING

Gas poisoning may be accidental or suicidal and possibly complicated by the effects of sleeping drugs. Gas most commonly found domestically is either natural or manufactured town gas. The use of the latter has diminished.

Natural gas causes asphyxia by diluting the available oxygen but it does not affect the blood haemoglobin. Being highly inflammable, if it accumulates in an enclosed space, there is a risk of explosion, even at fairly low concentrations.

Manufactured town gas causes haemoglobin to unite with carbon monoxide in the gas, thereby preventing the normal combination of the haemoglobin with oxygen.

In both cases the brain is deprived of its oxygen supply and, if the condition is severe or prolonged, the respiratory centre of the brain ceases to work, breathing stops and death follows. Resuscitation must be initiated without delay if breathing is shallow or imperceptible.

The situation in which the casualty is discovered will be a major factor in deciding the need for resuscitation.

**Do not use a naked light in the presence of gas.**

SIGNS AND SYMPTOMS

Those poisoned by town gas may be a cherry-red colour; those, by natural gas a normal pink or a cyanosed, blue colour.

TREATMENT

Treatment is directed to keeping the blood as fully oxygenated as possible by maintaining adequate ventilation.

The casualty should be removed into fresh air to help disperse the gas in his lungs and lessen any risk of injury from explosion.

Resuscitation should be initiated clear of the contaminated air.

It is vital to draw well clear between breaths to avoid contamination from the casualty's exhaled air.

**NB** Because the only gas present (provided you do not remain in the contaminated area) is that in the casualty's lungs, the first-aider should not be overcome herself by the victim's exhaled air.

Whenever possible, pure oxygen should be given by intermittent positive pressure. This is much better than air, but is seldom available at once.

*Recovery*

Recovery from the effects of gas poisoning is much slower than that from the effects of near-drowning. Resuscitation may have to be continued for a much longer period before normal breathing is restored.

## Other forms of poisoning similar to gas

The effects of gas poisoning and its treatment have been mentioned separately, but the same instructions apply to poisoning arising from the exhaust fumes of a car, inefficient ventilation from a defective heater and from stoves, particularly coke stoves, used without adequate ventilation.

All instances are essentially carbon monoxide poisoning. Carbon monoxide itself is odourless, but there may be fumes from other substances present.

SIGNS AND SYMPTOMS

People poisoned in these ways may experience giddiness, drowsiness, faintness, palpitation and nausea. They will recover in fresh air.

## Gases other than carbon monoxide

There are a variety of circumstances which may lead to fatalities; all ultimately involve lack of oxygenation of the blood supply. Common examples are:

### Irritant fumes

Irritant fumes produce inflammation of the lungs, which results in inadequate oxygen transfer and an eventual failure of respiration. At this stage resuscitation is needed, preferably with the added administration of pure oxygen if available.

These circumstances may arise in industrial accidents, when, for example, ammonia containers burst.

### Manufactured poisonous gases

Some gases are manufactured as poisons; for example, Cyanogen which is used for killing vermin and which poisons the nervous system very quickly.

### Carbon dioxide

Carbon dioxide is normally present in the air in minute concentration and a function of the respiratory system is to remove it from the body. However, a concentration of carbon dioxide will have a paralysing effect on the respiratory centre of the brain. Death can occur rapidly in exposure to a high concentration.

**Sewer gas and mine gas**

The picture may be a mixed one and include a lack of oxygen, poisoning by carbon dioxide, methane, carbon monoxide and sulphuretted hydrogen.

**Oxygen lack**

Lack of oxygen occurs in places which are not ventilated or not opened up for long intervals. Examples are double bottoms of ships and underground tanks.

In such compartments it is possible for the oxygen in the enclosed air to be absorbed by painted surfaces or to be used up in the rusting of metallic surfaces.

Immediate resuscitation in fresh air is vital.

Compartments such as these should be entered only by rescuers wearing breathing apparatus with an air or oxygen supply.

A handerchief over the nose or a 'gas mask' gives no protection against oxygen lack, carbon monoxide or carbon dioxide.

*Follow-up care*

The follow-up care of all victims of poisoning is vital. Supportive or symptomatic treatment should be carried out as necessary and is as important as other aspects of therapy. There may be lack of oxygen or fluids. The patient may be in shock (see pages 58–62) or if he or she has attempted suicide, in a critical emotional state. These and other related symptoms should be given attention after the drug or gas has been neutralised or removed.

## OTHER POISONS FOUND IN THE HOME

While the commonest cause of home-poisonings is by coal gas, there are other possible poisons in many homes. Barbiturates and aspirin are the two which readily spring to mind, as so many people take sleeping pills or pain-relievers. But the number of possible poisonings in the home is increasing all the time, chiefly with the widespread use of insecticides and weedkillers. Household cleansers and polishes are also a hazard, especially where there are young children about.

The action in all cases is to treat the state of shock and remove the patient to hospital at once. If possible, determine the poison taken—effects vary. The following are but examples:

### Acids

Battery acid—sulphuric acid—is very poisonous. It is colourless and if kept in a bottle can be mistaken for glycerine. It is very corrosive and will burn the mouth and tongue. It will also cause great pain. Collapse and shock will occur and must be treated immediately and on the way to medical aid.

### Alkalies

Caustic soda can be mistaken for salts and taken as a laxative. This is why all such substances *must* be stored in a labelled bottle. Caustic soda will cause swelling of the lips and tongue and burning pain from mouth to stomach. Retching and vomiting will occur. Shock is usually severe and will need to be treated at once.

Ammonia is another poison often stored in the home. If fumes get into the eyes they can cause severe irritation and the eyes must be flushed out at once. As both eyes are usually affected, the quickest method is to plunge the face into a bowl of tepid water.

### Antihistamines

Children may mistake some antihistamines for sweets. Although obtainable without prescription, antihistamines should be kept in a locked cupboard.

The most common effects of an overdose are drowsiness or sleep but there may be giddiness, headache, dry mouth and even vomiting and diarrhoea. If a large overdose has been taken, breathing may cease and artificial respiration will be required.

### Aspirin

The fatal dose of aspirin varies. Moderately toxic doses cause nausea and tinnitis. Deafness can also occur. If larger doses are taken, there will be mental confusion, drowsiness or coma. The patient will sweat profusely and may vomit some blood.

A stomach washout is usually necessary.

## Barbiturates

There is a great variety of barbiturates, but they can be roughly divided into those which act quickly but last a short time, and those which act more slowly for a longer period. Some sleeping capsules contain both ingredients.

When a poisonous dose has been taken, the first effects are giddiness, instability and headache. The victim falls asleep but this may be preceded by a period of excitable talk and action. Sometimes there is cyanosis, especially around the lips. Breathing may be noisy. Pupils are small but not pin-point as with morphine poisoning.

## Insecticides

Many insecticides are poisonous and all shall be stored and used with great care.

DDT is fairly harmless unless a large quantity is swallowed. It causes aching in the limbs, muscular weakness and sometimes convulsions.

Gammexane produces the same symptoms.

Strychnine is sometimes used for killing moles. As it is a very dangerous poison it should never be kept on household premises. Poisoning by strychnine causes very intense pain and muscular spasms.

## Iron

Because iron tablets are often an attractive colour, children sometimes mistake them for sweets. A large quantity can be dangerous. The child will become pale and vomit (sometimes blood). Shock, drowsiness and restlessness may develop.

## Lead

Acute lead poisoning is rare. Chronic poisoning (most often seen in children who have bitten or sucked articles such as railings, paint or toys containing lead) results in drowsiness, irritability, headache, insomnia, loss of appetite, constipation and colicky pain.

## Lysol

Lysol is a corrosive poison, causing burning of the tongue and mouth. Although initially there is pain, this disappears after a time as lysol has an anaesthetic effect.

The victim will collapse, become unconscious, and is likely to vomit; it is especially important to see that this is not inhaled. The victim should be treated in the recovery position (Fig. 32).

## Mercury

Some seed-dressings and insecticides contain mercury. The first symptoms of poisoning will be irritation, and a 'feeling of heat' in the throat. There will also be faintness and vomiting. Later, severe abdominal pain will occur and, much later, diarrhoea.

It is important to differentiate between food poisoning and metallic poisonings. Whereas in food poisoning vomiting stops fairly soon, in mercury (and arsenic) poisoning, it will continue. In food poisoning, diarrhoea begins early but in mercury and arsenic poisoning it may be delayed for as long as 12 hours.

## Paraffin

Paraffin and petrol are sometimes swallowed accidentally by children. The immediate effect is restlessness, vomiting and diarrhoea. The victim may become drowsy or fit or both.

## Weedkillers

Arsenic is often present in weedkillers, horticultural sprays, powders for destroying ants and other similar preparations in household use. The storage and use of all these should be undertaken with great care.

Arsenic is tasteless. Symptoms of arsenic poisoning are similar to those of mercury poisoning.

Sodium chlorate is the least harmful weedkiller for general use. Those containing paraquat are safe if the given instructions are carefully observed. If accidentally drunk, headache, tight chest pains and sensitivity to light (photophobia) will result. Sometimes the victim's kidneys become affected.

### Wintergreen

Oil of wintergreen is intended for external use, but the smell sometimes tempts children to drink it. As the active principle is salicylate the symptoms and treatment are the same as those for aspirin poisoning.

## POISONING BY PLANTS

Aconite is the poison found in monkshood, often grown in gardens. It is also contained in aconite liniment, which may be taken accidentally. It is one of the most powerful poisons known. Its effect and those of other

**Table 2** Signs and symptoms of plant poisoning

| Name of plant | Part which is poisonous | Signs/symptoms of poisoning |
|---|---|---|
| Aconite | All parts especially seeds and roots | Tightening and burning of mouth and skin. Sickness, loose stools, fits, twitching, collapse. |
| Berberis | Berries | Purging. |
| Broom | Only the leaves are poisonous | Burning in mouth, sickness, loose stools, fits and twitchings. |
| Cherry | Stones if broken and chewed | General weakness, heaviness of arms and legs, increasing difficulty in breathing, headache, dizziness, sickness, watering of the eyes, irritation of the throat. |
| Daffodil | Bulb | Sickness and loose stools. |
| Deadly nightshade | Berries | Confusion, excitability, flushed face, dry mouth, dilated pupils giving a startled appearance, rapid pulse rate. |

*continued overleaf*

**Table 2** *continued*

| Name of plant | Part which is poisonous | Signs/symptoms of poisoning |
|---|---|---|
| Elderberry | Leaves and bark | As for broken cherry stones. |
| Hemlock | Seeds | Rapid breathing, slow pulse rate, dilated pupils, paralysis. |
| Holly | Berries | Sickness, loose stools, sleepiness. |
| Hydrangea | All parts | As for broken cherry stones. |
| Laburnum | All parts (Britain's second most poisonous tree). When ripe, poison is concentrated in the seeds, pods and leaves | Burning in mouth, sickness, loose stools, exhaustion, mental confusion, fits leading to coma. |
| Lupin | Seeds especially. Other parts to a lesser extent | Shallow breathing, twitchings, paralysis, fits leading to collapse. |
| Marihuana | Leaves | Stimulation of senses, hallucinations, blurred vision, sleepiness, difficulty in walking. |
| Mistletoe | All parts but the berries especially | Sickness, loose stools, slow pulse rate. |
| Narcissus | Bulbs | Sickness and loose stools. |
| Thornapple | Seeds | As for deadly nightshade. |
| Yew | All parts. Seeds especially poisonous. *This is Britain's most poisonous tree* | Severe stomach pain, sickness, loose stools, paralysis, fits. Death if not dealt with within five minutes. |

plants are shown in Table 2. The first symptom is numbness followed by tingling of the mouth. Later it gives rise to very profuse salivation, pains in the head and difficulty in swallowing. A prickling sensation of the skin is typical and does not occur with other poisons. This poison can cause death very quickly. Medicinal powdered charcoal, if available, may act as an antidote, and if the patient can swallow, may be given in tablespoonfuls mixed with water or milk.

## Belladonna

Belladonna is the active principle of deadly nightshade. This plant has black, shiny berries and should not be confused with the red berried woody nightshade, which is only very slightly poisonous. It is, of course, also found in belladonna liniments, and is sometimes included in indigestion mixtures.

Most cases of belladonna poisoning do recover. Belladonna causes a very dry mouth with no saliva, difficulty in swallowing and a hoarse voice. The pupils are so widely dilated that the coloured iris nearly disappears. The skin is flushed and dry and there can be a pink rash. The patient may be excited and even delirious.

## Colchicum

The active principle, colchicine, is found in the Autumn crocus. This poison does not act at once, but after several hours there are abdominal pains, vomiting and diarrhoea.

## Hemlock

Sometimes grown in gardens, hemlock contains coniine. This causes burning of the mouth and throat, drowsiness, staggering, and difficulty in breathing. Artificial respiration may be needed.

## Laburnum

Children may eat the fallen pods and seeds from the decorative laburnum tree. Symptoms of laburnum poisoning do not appear at once. Some hours later there may be vomiting, tachycardia, dilated pupils and dizziness.

## POISONING BY MARINE LIFE

Contact with marine animals can produce puncture-wounds (usually on the hands and feet) as well as toxic reactions. These reactions vary greatly, depending upon individual sensitivity or resistance and on the virulence and amount of venom contacted.

Jellyfish and Portuguese man-of-war have stinging cells—nematocysts—on their tentacles which discharge venom through threadlike tubes on contact, producing burning pain and a rash with very small haemorrhages in the skin. Sometimes the victim becomes shocked, and experiences muscular cramping, nausea and vomiting and respiratory difficulty. Tentacles may cling to the victim's skin, when they should be gently removed with a towel and the area washed thoroughly with diluted ammonia. Aspirin, or something similar, for the relief of pain may be given.

Stingrays inflict lacerations or punctures and inject toxic venom from glandular tissue that is an integral part of their caudal spine. General symptoms include shock, vomiting, diarrhoea, and muscular paralysis. First aid consists of soaking the wounds in hot water (heat may help to inactivate the venom); the control of bleeding and the application of dry dressings. Medical aid should be sought at once as the wound will require thorough cleansing and removal of fragments of the stingray's spine.

## SNAKE BITES

In Britain and many European countries, the common snake is the adder, whose bite is but moderately venomous. The creature tends to live in mountainous areas, moorlands and clearings or the edges of woodlands and forested areas.

The harmless grass snake has a streamlined appearance ending in a tapered head. Its markings are rows of dark spots and a yellow-orange band between the eyes. The smooth snake is also harmless, is the same length as the adder but has a thinner head; its grey (occasionally brown) body has rows of paired dots and the flush set of its scales give it a smooth skin.

If the snake is poisonous fang and teeth marks will show on the skin (Fig. 72), non-poisonous bites would result in teeth marks only (Fig. 73).

It is the adder's bite which is painful. Sometimes the area or even the whole affected limb becomes swollen and bruised. This can be alarming. General reactions include sweating, vomiting and diarrhoea. Stomach pains or loss of consciousness are very rare.

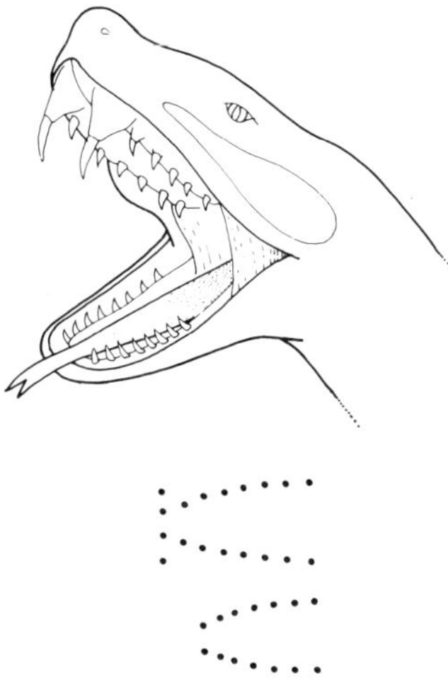

**Fig. 72** Poisonous snake bite showing fang marks.

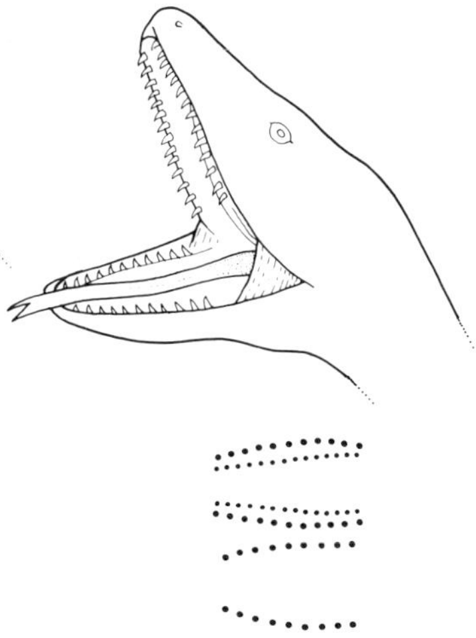

**Fig. 73** Non-poisonous snake bite showing teeth marks only.

First aid consists of complete rest. Immobilise the bitten part immediately and treat as if fractured. This prevents, or slows down, the spread of poison. Reassure the victim by telling him that this is the most he will suffer. Cover the bite with a dry dressing. Aspirin or a similar pain reliever may help until medical aid is available.

## ANIMAL BITES

The bite of any animal, whether wild, in a zoo or a pet, may result in an open wound. Dog and cat bites are common. The principal danger of animal bites is rabies. Warm blooded animals such as dogs, cats, bats, racoons and rabbits can transmit the rabies virus through their saliva by means of biting the victim or by licking the individual on abraded skin. Contrary to popular belief, the animal need not be drooling, irritable or appear dangerous. In some cases, the animal will appear partially paralysed, stuporous, quiet or even affectionate. The most common sites involved are the limbs. Bites around the head, neck and face areas are considered to be more serious because of a shorter incubation period.

An animal in the final stages of rabies infection will usually develop symptoms of the disease and die within a few days of symptomatic infection.

The human incubation period for rabies varies considerably but averages around 2 months. The diagnosis of rabies is based on the history of contact, laboratory studies of the animal and the presence of clinical symptoms in the animal (when the creature is available). The disease is virtually always fatal in man once the symptoms have appeared. The total course of the symptomatic disease is about 7 days. As the total course of survival is long (24–155 days from the time of the bite) however, there is usually time to treat the victim and prevent the symptomatic onset of the disease. The first aid treatment consists of washing the wound with large quantities of soap and water. Keep the part immobile. If available, apply a dry dressing and bandage it in position. Seek medical attention promptly.

Restrain the animal if possible.

The police should also be called to help. If the animal has to be killed, the brain should not be injured as it will be needed for study to confirm viral rabies infection.

## MINOR BITES AND STINGS

For minor bites and stings—including nettle stings which can cause distress to children—cold applications may be used and soothing lotions, such as calamine, may bring some relief.

A combination of poison mortality rates and related statistics are gathered in Appendix 3.

## NURSES' RESPONSIBILITIES IN RELATION TO DRUGS

The care, custody and administration of today's multiplicity of drugs represent great responsibilities for nurses.

Mistakes can occur in the prescribing, the dispensing, the labelling and the interpretation of instructions, as well as in the actual administration of a drug. It is important, therefore, not only that nurses adhere closely to laid down procedures themselves but that they also ensure that all with whom they work employ safe techniques in any procedure which involves the use of drugs.

### In hospital

In hospital, although the pharmacist is responsible for the storage, labelling and distribution of drugs throughout the building, the care, custody and administration of drugs in a ward or department are the responsibility of the sister or charge nurse. This responsibility may be delegated only in accordance with the employing authority's policy which should be formulated in consultation with all the staff involved.

All drugs should be kept in a locked cupboard and the key held by the sister or charge nurse or whomsoever has been designated by the employing authority. Medicine trolleys containing individual prescriptions and stock items, when not in use should either be secured to a wall by a locking device or kept inside a locked cupboard or room. Drugs should be carried in locked containers when being transported within the hospital building.

No drug should be administered by a nurse without a written prescription except in times of real emergencies. Only a trained nurse should accept a verbal order and only if she or he *fully* understands the total prescription. When a patient is required to take drugs after being discharged from hospital, it is vital to ascertain before leaving the ward that the patient understands the drug schedule, possible side effects and any special safeguards that should be taken, such as the avoidance of drinking alcohol, eating certain foods or driving a motor vehicle.

### In the community

Drugs prescribed by the patient's general practitioner or supplied by the hospital's pharmaceutical department and given to the patient on discharge, are the patient's own property and will be kept by him or her. The community nurse, however, should check that the patient fully understands his or her drug regimen and the necessity of safe storage of all drugs and medicines.

Sometimes the community psychiatric nurse is required to keep a patient's drugs and to administer them in accordance with the prescription. The drugs should then be kept in a locked cupboard or safe in the nurse's own home. When transporting such drugs by motor car they should be placed either in a lockable glove compartment or the boot.

## Controlled drugs

Controlled drugs must be kept in a locked safe or other receptacle with a warning light to show when the door is open.

### Administration of drugs

The actual administration of drugs is a nursing responsibility. Useful information and guidance on this subject can be found in two short publications of the Royal College of Nursing:

*Drug Administration: a Nursing Responsibility.*

*The Duties and Responsibilities of Occupational Health Nurses Under the Provisions of the Medicines Act 1968 and Subsequent Regulations.* (Leaflet 11.)

### The Medicines Act 1968

The Acts which currently relate to drugs in usual medical practice are the Misuse of Drugs Act 1971 and the Medicines Act 1968 with Statutory Instruments 1977 (1243) and 1979 (299).

CHAPTER 11

# Emergencies in the Home: Prevention and Care

The word *home* conjures up a place of comfort and security, and most people feel safer in their own homes than anywhere else. But the reality of the situation is different. Every year in the United Kingdom the number of deaths due to accidents in the home almost equals the number of deaths due to accidents on the roads. In each case the number is not inconsiderable.

In 1976 for example, 6407 people died from home accidents, whilst 6570 were killed on the roads. Furthermore, there are more non-fatal accidents in the home than on the roads; so many homes are far from safe. The salutary fact is that a very high proportion of accidents in the home are preventable, so why are they not prevented?

In many cases, householders do not seriously consider the matter of home safety. It is only after the accident has occurred that one hears the phrase 'I never thought . . .'; tragic words when spoken after the death of a loved child in a home accident. Often a little imagination and a reasonable amount of common sense (which incidentally is not very common!) is all that is needed to make the home a real place of safety.

The two ages which are most vulnerable to accidents are the extremes of life—the very young and the very old. Young children are naturally curious and do not realise the dangers of, for instance, fire and electricity. So if there are children in the house, action must be taken to make the home safer for them. Old people are often frail and find walking difficult; eyesight and hearing may be impaired, so again the environment must be assessed to make sure that the elderly are safe. Over half the accidents in the home which result in death are falls; about three quarters of these occur in people over 65 years of age. This demonstrates quite clearly the main area of danger for old people. An increasing number of people move to sheltered housing accommodation when they grow old. These units are carefully designed to reduce the risk of falls, but much can be done to minimise the danger in any home.

One chapter cannot provide an exhaustive guide to the whole subject of home accidents. This attempts therefore to draw attention to the most common types of accident, to suggest the lines of prevention and to indicate the first aid treatment when accidents do occur.

## FALLS

There is a wide variety of causes of falls (see also pages 82–5 for care of patients with fractures). Small children do not have a very sound sense of balance and therefore fall over very easily. While restrictions must not be allowed to affect their normal development a reasonable amount of care will ensure that they do not hurt themselves when they do tumble. Injuries will result if children fall from a height, so precautions should be taken to prevent them climbing on to chairs and tables. Toddlers should play inside a play-pen and only be out of it when an adult is with them (Fig. 74a). Gates across the top and bottom of flights of stairs are necessary until the child can manage to go up and down stairs safely (Fig. 74b). Garden swings and climbing frames give great pleasure, but small children should not be allowed to play on them alone; an adult or a responsible older child should be present.

As children grow older they tend to get more adventurous and it

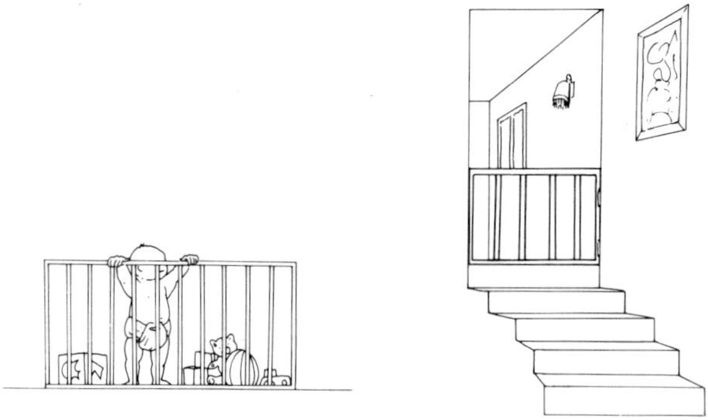

(a) (b)

**Fig. 74** Safety in the home: (a) toddler in a playpen and (b) gate at the top of the stairs.

seems impossible to keep them out of mischief (Fig. 75a). Whilst encouraging normal development, parents should impress safety measures on their children and ensure that there are no obvious hazards. A ladder left against a wall, for example, is a frank invitation to a child to climb it; similarly, an open loft door presents exciting possibilities.

As far as adults are concerned, falls in the home are usually due to either tripping over something on the floor or failing to observe adequate precautions when reaching up to a shelf or cupboard. Floor coverings must be kept in good repair; worn patches in carpets, holes and tears in linoleum or vinyl are all dangerous. Wooden floors should have a non-slip finish and polish must never be applied under rugs or mats. Articles should not be left on the floor and dogs and cats should be trained to lie and sleep only in their baskets out of harm's way. Adequate lighting is important, so that people can see where they are

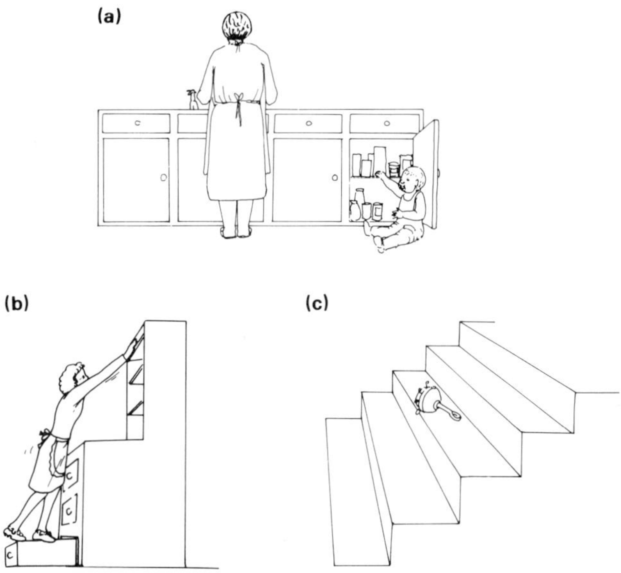


**Fig. 75** Dangers in the home: (a) housewife at the sink while her toddler investigates the cupboard; (b) housewife standing on an open drawer and (c) a child's toy left on the stairs.

treading. It is a relief to take shoes off when at home, but floppy mules or slippers should not be worn all the time; a pair of soft shoes is just as comfortable, and much safer.

When cleaning, or working at home, people frequently have to stretch up for things that are out of reach. Falls often occur because individuals are careless. A housewife wants a dish out of a high cupboard in the kitchen and as she is in a hurry she pulls out a drawer and stands on it (Fig. 75b); someone painting the bathroom cannot quite reach the far corner and stands on the bath edge; someone else kneels on a narrow window-sill to clean the top of the window; just three examples of situations which can result in very nasty falls. Every home should have a pair of small, light steps which are easily carried about and people should get into the habit of always using them.

Old people are especially prone to falls. Indeed everyday in the United Kingdom, an average of 8 old people die from this one cause. Special care must be taken in any home where there are elderly people. All the foregoing points are applicable to them and it should always be remembered that many elderly people have poor sight, so they cannot see the hazards which are obvious to younger members of the family. Floors must be kept free from extraneous articles like toys, brushes and tools, and electric flex should not be trailed across the floor (Fig. 75c). The bathroom and lavatory should be adapted for safety, with grab rails and handles by the bath and on the wall by the lavatory seat. A non-slip mat in the bath is a useful precautionary measure.

## TREATMENT

The first aid treatment for those injured in falls obviously varies with the extent and type of injury, but there are certain basic principles to follow in every case. It should not be forgotten that adults, especially elderly ones, may have fallen because of a medical emergency, for example, a stroke, so there may be more to deal with than just the fall.

As always, the first action is to ensure that the casualty is breathing and has a clear airway. The first-aider should then assess the situation and no attempt should be made to move the victim until this has been done. Every person who has fallen suffers a certain amount of shock and this is increased by efforts to stand up again immediately. If the casualty is conscious and there seems no obvious injury, after a few minutes he or she can be helped to a nearby chair, bed or settee and allowed to rest until he or she has recovered from shock.

If the casualty is unconscious, it is vital that the first-aider ensures that the airway is clear. An ambulance should be called, the patient kept warm but not overheated; no attempt should be made to move the patient if the ambulance is expected within a short time, as the ambulance crew will lift the patient on to a stretcher and straight into the ambulance. If the house is isolated, or very bad weather means a long delay before the arrival of the ambulance, and there is help to hand, it may be practicable to move the patient to a bed, settee or a more convenient place on the floor.

If the casualty is conscious, and complaining of a severe pain in a leg or arm, it is possible that a bone has been fractured. Under these circumstances, it is always wise to treat the patient as if a fracture has occurred. An ambulance should be called. Whilst waiting for its arrival, the first-aider may be able to make the patient more comfortable. The injured limb should be handled as little as possible and if attempts to move the patient cause increased pain, matters should be left alone. An injured leg can be tied to the sound leg; this will effectively immobilise the fracture.

Falling forwards on to the hand may result in a fracture of the wrist. The forearm should be supported by a folded newspaper which is bandaged into position (Fig. 76a) before putting the arm in a large arm sling (Fig. 76b). If there is pain in the elbow or upper arm, the whole arm should be bandaged to the patient's body. The aim of any first aid is to immobilise the area in order to prevent further damage. If it is doubtful whether there is any injury other than bruising after a fall, it is always wise to err on the side of caution. Persistent pain, increased swelling or inability to move freely or properly are warning signs which must not be disregarded.

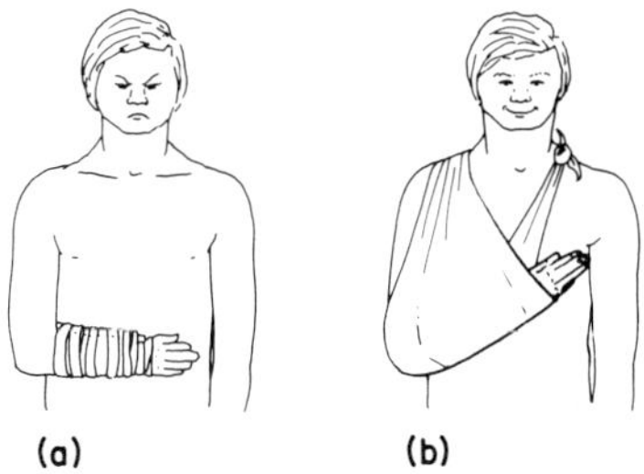

(a) (b)

**Fig. 76** Immobilisation of a fractured wrist: (a) forearm supported by a folded newspaper and (b) arm enclosed in a sling.

HOSPITAL MANAGEMENT

On arrival in hospital, the patient will be X-rayed and if a fracture has occurred, the break will be set and the limb immobilised. An anaesthetic may be necessary for this, and therefore no patient with a suspected fracture should be given anything to eat or drink.

## CUTS AND LACERATIONS

There are very few days in life when people do not handle knives, scissors or other cutting implements, so cuts and lacerations are common injuries. Fortunately most of them are minor, but almost all can be prevented if proper care is taken.

Many cooks pride themselves on the sharpness of their kitchen and carving knives; these knives are not usually jumbled up in a drawer because this spoils the cutting edge. Kitchen knives should be kept in a proper rack, either in separate slots or held magnetically and well out of the way of small children. Knives should be used only for the purpose for which they are intended and used with care on a flat surface. Accidents are almost inevitable if sharp knives are used to lever off bottle tops or open parcels. Children should be taught from an early age to use knives properly, only for their correct use, and with care.

The same applies to scissors. Good dressmaking scissors, for instance, should be kept in the work box and used only for cutting materials. Children who want to cut out scraps or shapes should be given special scissors with rounded ends, which cut paper well but are unlikely to damage the child's fingers. Scissors with sharp points should never be handled by small children, as they cause dangerous puncture wounds if driven into the body. They may also result in loss of sight if they penetrate the eye.

Other objects with sharp edges are often found in the tool box and garden shed. Saws, chisels and knives should be kept in a safe and secure place, well out of the reach of small children. Again, they should be used properly and only for their intended purpose. Lawn mowers, garden shears and secateurs must be used with care and never left in places where the unwary can trip over them or accidentally walk onto the blades. Especial care must be taken with electrically or motor driven mowers or shears. The blades must never be handled when the machine is switched on; tips or parts of fingers can be lost in a split second if the blades start moving. This danger seems obvious; but every summer claims a number of casualties, who, when mowing the lawn, bend down to probe a stone or clod of earth out of the blades, without first switching off the power.

Accidents which involve objects with a cutting edge usually cause incised wounds, but lacerated wounds can be caused by such things as a protruding nail. A house which is well maintained is unlikely to contain such hazards, but fences, garden sheds and gates may be the site of such dangerous snags.

Cracked or chipped crockery and glass are more likely to break than sound articles, and some very unpleasant wounds can result if breakages occur when one of these objects is being handled. It can be seen that in homes which are kept tidy and in good order the risk of sustaining a wound is reduced to a minimum. However, in spite of all precautions, accidents may occur.

## Clean incised wounds

With a clean incised wound, as soon as the skin is broken, blood starts to escape immediately.

### TREATMENT

The first treatment of wounds is *to stop the bleeding.* Blood will eventually clot of its own accord, and the aim is to help this natural process. What is actually done is influenced by the amount and rate of blood loss.

If the wound is a small one, pressure over it will help to arrest bleeding in a very short time. The skin around the area should be washed clean and then a dressing applied.

A larger wound will bleed more freely and require more urgent treatment. The casualty should sit or lie down with the injured part raised above heart level. The edges of the wound should be brought together and pressure maintained on the area for about 10 minutes. As soon as the blood flow diminishes, a dressing, clean handkerchief or clean piece of linen should be placed over the wound.

When the bleeding has stopped, the skin surrounding the area should be gently cleansed; it must be remembered that a newly formed blood clot can easily be dislodged and if this happens, bleeding will start again. The clean dressing should be bandaged firmly into place.

If further oozing occurs, the original dressing should not be removed. Pressure should be applied over it and then another dressing to cover it. If the loss of blood is severe, the patient may need further treatment in hospital. Wounds of this severity will probably need stitching and even a blood transfusion may be required.

Throughout the whole incident, the casualty must be reassured. Most people are very frightened when they see their own blood flowing away; reassurance comes from a confident first-aider behaving in a calm and assured manner.

## Lacerations

A laceration is a tear in the skin and its underlying tissues; bleeding may not be as severe as that from an incised wound, but the damage to tissues may be just as great. Lacerated wounds are often difficult to assess, especially if they are dirty.

TREATMENT

They should be washed, if possible under running water. If there is anything embedded in the wound, such as a piece of garden cane or sliver of glass, the casualty should receive medical attention as soon as possible. A dressing applied directly over the wound will drive the foreign body further in, so a ring bandage should be applied. This is made by twisting a bandage or piece of cloth into a ring which is then placed to surround the wound; pressure on it will help to arrest bleeding (Fig. 77). This ring should be bandaged in place before the patient is taken to hospital or to the doctor's surgery.

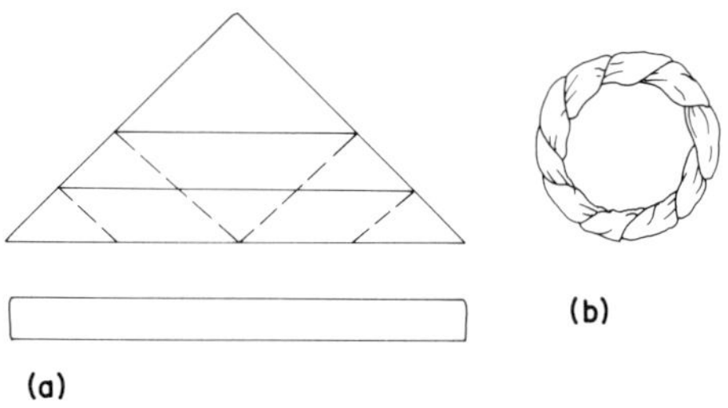


**Fig. 77** Formation of a ring pad showing (a) a folded triangle and (b) ends tied together after twisting to form a ring.

If there is no foreign body in the wound, it should be washed thoroughly and a dressing applied. Lacerated wounds are more prone to sepsis than incised ones and for a few days after injury signs of sepsis should be watched for. If the patient develops pain, and the area becomes swollen and red, medical advice should be sought without delay.

## ASPHYXIA (SUFFOCATION)

Suffocation means that air is not reaching the lungs, a state of affairs which will rapidly lead to death unless it is treated promptly (see also pages 130–1). The main causes of suffocation in the home are:

- mechanical blockage of the air passages, as in choking or when a plastic bag is over the nose and mouth
- replacement of air by some other substance, that is, water, as in drowning, or carbon monoxide, as in a closed garage with the car engine running
- failure of the nervous system to initiate respiration, as in electrocution

### GENERAL PRINCIPLES OF TREATMENT

Act at once.

*Either*

Remove the cause from the patient, for example, a polythene bag over the head, a cord around the neck and the like. If the victim is buried, clear earth, sand or snow away at least down to the waist so that the chest can move to allow breathing.

Hook out with the finger, false teeth or food which are obstructing the airway.

For sudden choking, give several hard thumps between the shoulder blades. (A child may be held upside down whilst this is done.)

*or*

Move the patient from the cause, for example, out of the water or from a fume-ladened atmosphere. (If there are fumes or smoke, breathe deeply before entering the room and then hold your breath for as long as possible while inside the room.)

Clear air passages and hold the jaw in position.

If patient is not breathing, begin resuscitation at once. When this has been successful, place him in the recovery position.

## Mechanical blockage of the air passages

### Choking

Nearly everyone has had experience of food 'going the wrong way', so the sensation of choking is known to most people. The victim is instantly aware that something is wrong and he starts to cough. A piece of food, a sweet or even a small denture, has been inhaled and has lodged at the top of the trachea. The airway is obstructed and as air cannot enter the lungs, the victim's colour changes, first to red and then to blue. Violent coughing is usually sufficient to dislodge the obstruction, but two or three sharp blows between the shoulder blades may assist this process. If it does not, further action must be taken promptly.

TREATMENT

If the victim is an adult, he or she should be told to stand up. The first-aider then stands close behind the victim and clasps her or his arms around the victim's chest, putting the hands one on top of the other, at the base of the victim's sternum in the space between the ribs. The first-aider should then give the victim a violent hug, bringing her or his hands in as far as possible. This will force the obstruction out, like a cork coming out of a bottle (Fig. 13, page 28).

This manoeuvre cannot be carried out on a baby or small child. An infant must be held upside down quickly and a child put over the first-aider's knees and struck between its shoulders (see page 27). Sometimes the cause of the obstruction can be hooked out of the mouth with the fingers. Fingers should not be put down the throat however—the obstruction can be pushed further in.

### Plastic bag over the nose and mouth

Many plastic bags carry clearly printed warnings about their danger, whilst others are perforated so that they are not airtight. In spite of this, they are the cause of a number of fatalities each year. Great care must be taken to see that small children cannot get hold of plastic bags to use them as 'space helmets' and the like. If, in spite of all precautions, a child does do this, the bag must be taken off quickly and artificial respiration started immediately (see page 20). Once normal breathing has been restored, the child should be kept quiet and seen by a doctor as soon as possible.

## Drowning

Drowning is not usually thought of as an accident in the home, but in fact it is not necessary to have a large amount of water in which to drown—a garden pond or a bath are often quite deep enough. The people to whom this accident is most likely to occur are small children, old people and adults who faint or fall from some other condition, for example, an epileptic fit.

Garden ponds should be wired over or securely fenced in, if there are children around. A small curious child investigating the goldfish, for instance, can drown in a matter of minutes when an adult's back is turned.

Old people should, ideally, take baths only when there is someone else in the house and the bathroom door should not be locked. A non-slip bath mat is useful; so is a grab rail or a handle by the bath; these enable elderly people to move with greater confidence. Adults who suffer from epilepsy are usually well aware of the potential dangers of their condition and act accordingly.

### TREATMENT

The victim must be moved from the water immediately. A child lifted out of a pond should be held upside down in order to drain as much water out of the lungs as possible. Any weeds or vegetation in the mouth must be removed and artificial respiration started immediately (see Chap. 2). As soon as breathing is established, the wet clothes should be stripped off, the child wrapped in a blanket and kept warm and quiet until full recovery.

If someone has drowned in the bath, the first-aider should pull out the plug and lift the victim's face out of the water. It is impossible to lift an unconscious person out of the bath unaided, so artificial respiration should be started with the casualty in the bath. This is easier said than done, and which method of resuscitation is used will be determined by the size and shape of the bath. Additional help will be required to lift the person out and on to the floor, where resuscitation must continue until breathing starts. The casualty should then be dried and kept warm and quiet in bed.

In all cases of resuscitation after drowning, the person should be seen by a doctor, preferably at home. When a first-aider's efforts at resuscitation are unsuccessful, the doctor and the police must be notified.

## Electrocution

Most homes contain a number of electrical appliances, which vary in size from coffee grinders, irons and razors, to washing machines, television sets and lawn mowers. Every appliance which is connected to the mains supply can be a potential danger under certain circumstances. Electricity is a good servant, but it can be a lethal master and must be treated with respect.

### Prevention

The wiring system of the house itself should be checked at intervals by a competent electrician; rewiring is costly, but expenditure of money in this instance may save a life. An adequate number of power points is essential, otherwise there is a temptation to run several appliances, such as the television set, a lamp, and a fire all off one plug. This overloading is not only dangerous in itself, but inevitably one or more of the appliances will have a long trailing flex, which is another hazard. Flex must be in good condition; frayed flex is dangerous and must be renewed immediately it becomes so (Fig. 78). Plugs also should be in good condition and wired up correctly.

The manufacturer's instructions about the use of equipment must be followed; this particularly applies to electric blankets and pads. Overblankets are designed to remain on whilst the user is in bed, but the

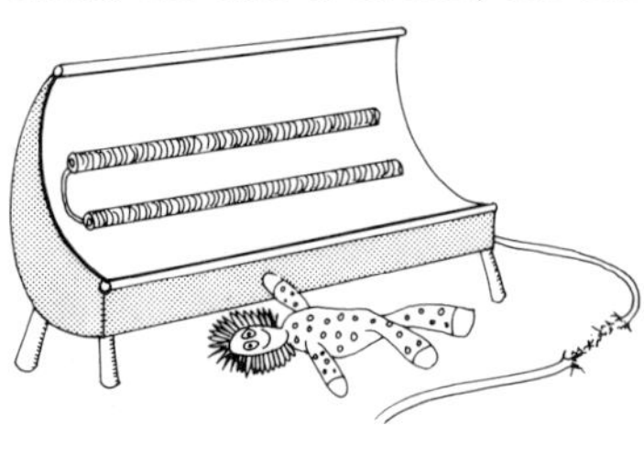

**Fig. 78** Three potential hazards of an electric fire: the frayed flex, the doll, dropped closely and touching, by the unguarded heated element.

majority of under blankets are not. An incontinent or sweating person in a bed with an electric underblanket switched on is in an absolutely lethal situation.

Bylaws now govern the way in which electricity is fitted into a bathroom, but many bathrooms were in use before these precautionary measures were introduced. As water and electricity form a potentially fatal combination, extra care must be taken when in the presence of both. Someone who has wet hands, or who is in the bath, is at very great risk if contact is made with an electrical object. Wall heaters and lights should have cord pulls, or be controlled by switches outside the bathroom. Electric shavers should only be used with properly insulated special sockets, and other electrical appliances should be kept out of the bathroom. Hair driers, for instance, should be used in the bedroom.

Power tools lighten work in the garden, but again must be treated with respect. Lawn mowers should not be used when the grass is wet and care must be taken not to mow the flex. Hedge cutters must be used according to the manufacturer's instructions and the flex kept well out of the way. Rubber soled shoes or rubber garden clogs will insulate the wearer, and it is a sensible precaution to wear these in the garden when using all power tools.

### TREATMENT

Anyone entering a room and finding someone lying on the floor, instinctively goes over and feels the pulse or turns them over to see what has happened. This action, if the casualty is electrically alive, that is attached to the source of the electricity, will result in two victims instead of one.

The current must be switched off, the plug pulled out of the socket or the cable wrenched free, before first aid can be given. Or, if this is not possible, standing on dry, insulating material (rubber, thickly folded newspaper, books or wood) and using similar material in your hands, knock or pull the patient clear of contact by using a walking stick, broom handle and the like if available.

Do not use an umbrella (it has metal ribs) and do not touch the victim with bare hands.

If, as is likely, breathing has stopped, and there is no sign of life, artificial respiration and cardiac massage must be started immediately. If there is someone else in the house, they should be asked to summon the doctor or an ambulance. If the first-aider is alone, and unable to attract the attention of a neighbour or passer by, resuscitation should continue until the victim recovers. If there are no signs of recovery after some time, the first-aider should dial 999 (or a similar emergency telephone call system) to summon help, then resume life saving measures until the ambulance arrives.

In all cases, an electrical burn is disregarded until the victim is breathing normally and has a steady pulse. Electrical burns can be deep and may require surgical treatment. Any first aid consists of covering the burn with a clean or sterile dressing until the patient reaches hospital, but this is of secondary importance. Unless the casualty is successfully resuscitated, the burn will be on a dead body—a situation of interest only to the coroner.

## FOREIGN BODIES

Foreign bodies in the eye or ear or skin of a patient are often more than just 'bothersome'; they can be distressingly painful. Careful and understanding treatment are required by the first-aider.

### TREATMENT: IN THE EYE

Instruct the patient not to rub the eye.

While the patient looks up, gently draw the lower lid down and out.

If the foreign body is seen on the lower lid, remove it with a moistened wisp of cotton wool or the corner of a clean handkerchief.

If the particle is thought to be under the upper lid, then, while the patient looks down, grasp the upper lid and draw it down and out over the lower lid. This should wipe away the foreign body. If not:

stand behind the patient

carefully place a smooth matchstick at the base of the upper lid; press it gently backwards

while the patient looks down, grasp the lashes of the upper lid to pull and evert it over the matchstick, remove particle as described above

**Do not** try to remove a foreign body from the eyeball or one which is embedded. Refer to a surgery.

TREATMENT: IN THE EAR

Turn the patient's head to the affected side: the object may drop out.

If an insect is inside the ear, lay the patient down with the affected ear uppermost. Pour in tepid water: the insect may float out.

If unsuccessful, refer to a surgery.

TREATMENT: IN THE SKIN

Fish hooks

Clean the wound area and the projecting part of the hook with soap and water.

**Do not** try to drag the intact hook back through the skin.

Push the point and the barb of the hook forward and through the skin.

Cut the barb.

Pull the remainder of the hook back through the skin.

Apply a dry dressing.

Refer to a surgery.

### The nose

In an adult, foreign bodies may enter the nose by accident but most commonly, the patient is a child who has inserted a bead or pea into the nostril. Attempts to remove this without an anaesthetic can be frightening and should be avoided.

TREATMENT

Instruct the casualty to breathe through the mouth.

Remove the casualty to hospital or to a surgery as soon as possible.

### The throat

Sensation arising from foreign bodies impacted above the level of the cricopharyngeus is usually referred to one side of the throat. Foreign bodies which the patient feels in the midline, however, are almost invariably impacted in the oesophagus, for this is the midline structure. They require oesophagoscopy for their removal.

The patient wearing an upper denture is not uncommonly the one who swallows a sizeable piece of bone, for the dental plate prevents detection of the foreign body by contact with the hard palate at the early stage when rejection is possible. By the time the patient feels the bone against the soft palate, the mechanism of deglutition has been initiated and it is too late to stop the bone being swallowed.

## POISONING

Because every home—and garden—contains a large number of substances which are dangerous if swallowed, aspects of poisoning are re-emphasised here (for a detailed coverage of the subject, see Chapter 10).

Adults recognise the danger and in any case have no desire to taste liquids such as bleach, ammonia, antifreeze, bubble bath, disinfectant, paint stripper or weedkiller. These and other liquids are often found, however, in places where they are accessible to children, and it is children who are usually the victims of this kind of poisoning. Obviously it is impractical to keep all bottles in locked cupboards, but in a home where there are children, parents should check the whereabouts of potentially dangerous substances and ensure that these are well out of the child's reach.

The majority of medicines are now dispensed in tablet form and bottles of these present another hazard. Parents are often conscientious about keeping the bathroom cabinet locked, but it is all too easy to overlook the bottle of pills kept on the bedside table or the mantelpiece. Some pills are dispensed in bottles with child-proof tops, but it is unwise to rely wholly on these. It is amazing what determined and inquisitive youngsters can open if they try.

Poisonous substances are also found in the garden (see Table 2, Chapter 10). Children are unlikely to chew rhubarb leaves or privet flowers, but some berries and seeds look like attractive sweets and are eaten as such. Laburnum seeds, honeysuckle berries, holly berries and the berries of common ivy are frequently found in gardens, whilst indoor plants such as the winter cherry or solanum also have attractive berries. All these and a number of other plants and trees are poisonous. Children, from a very early age, should be taught *never* to eat the berries, flowers or leaves of any plant unless an adult says they may do so.

Children are poisoned because they swallow substances without realising the danger, but adults may deliberately swallow overdoses of drugs or other toxic substances. Another danger is that sometimes people forget they have already taken a certain drug and swallow another dose; this is especially liable to happen at night. Someone takes a sleeping pill, goes to sleep for a short while, then wakes up. There is no recollection of having taken the first pill, so another one is taken, thus doubling the prescribed dosage. Drugs and alcohol together sometimes form a dangerous mixture; each on its own is not a poison, but taken together they can be.

A poisoning situation is often a confused situation, and it may be very difficult to establish just what has been swallowed. Children playing in a garden, for instance, cannot always say with certainty which berries they ate. Or even if they can identify them, they cannot say how many they swallowed. If a child gets hold of a bottle of tablets and swallows some, the number taken will also be unknown unless the owner remembers how many were in the bottle originally. So often all that can be said is that it seems likely that the child has swallowed an unknown amount of a substance which may, or may not, be identified.

### TREATMENT

It is always better to err on the side of caution, and seek medical advice, even if the child does not seem ill, as some poisons take a little while to manifest themselves. If signs of poisoning are present (for example, vomiting, drowsiness, convulsions, unconsciousness) speedy treatment is imperative and an ambulance should be called. The casualty should be placed in the recovery position (see Fig. 32) and the airway must be kept clear. It may be necessary to give artificial respiration. Any vomit should be saved and the bottle of tablets or a spray of the plant responsible for the poisoning should accompany the patient to hospital. If known, the time at which the poison was swallowed should be noted.

If the poison is a corrosive, the mouth and surrounding skin should be gently flushed with tepid water. Drinks of water may be given to a conscious patient. The corrosive may have spilled over the clothes, and if so, the affected area should be removed or cut away before the skin underneath is burned.

Following any case of poisoning, there may be various enquiries regarding the situation. The first-aider is therefore advised to make a note of the events at the time they happened and to retain these notes for further reference if questions are asked of her.

## BURNS AND SCALDS

The hazard of fire in the home is a serious one and householders should always be alert to this danger. Even a smouldering cigarette-end can start a fire which will quickly blaze through a house. Sensible precautions against such an occurrence should always be observed.

Fires, whether coal, gas or electric, should always be guarded if there is a child or a very old person in the house (Fig. 73). Guards must be adequate in size and fixed firmly in position. Some central heating radiators can get very hot and if they do, they also should be guarded. Especial care must be taken when using free-standing oil stoves. They should stand in a safe place, away from draughts, and should not be carried about when lighted.

Clothes made of inflammable material should not be bought for young children or old people. Billowing garments such as nightgowns are a more dangerous fire risk than pyjamas. By law, children's ready-made nightdresses must be manufactured from flame-resistant material for which there is a British Standard test.

A mirror should never be hung over a fireplace.

There is an element of risk in the kitchen whenever cooking is in progress. Saucepan handles must always be turned so that they cannot be accidentally knocked over or pulled down by children. Safety guards, which fit round the edge of the cooker and into which saucepan handles fit, are useful if there are children in the house.

Hot fat easily catches fire. If this happens, no attempt should be made to dowse the fire with water. The gas or electric ring must be turned off immediately and the pan covered with a large saucepan lid or an asbestos mat. If a chemical fire extinguisher is available, this can be used, or a fire blanket to smother the flames. As soon as the fire is put out, the pan should be left to cool where it is, as hot fat is liable to flare up again if it comes into contact with air. Boiling liquids must be handled carefully and small children should not be allowed to run about in the kitchen when pans are being moved off the stove.

Smokers must be careful and ash trays should be of adequate size. Special care should be taken at night before going to bed to check that there are no smouldering cigarette ends left in ash trays. Some people smoke in bed: this is dangerous and a practice which should be discouraged.

### TREATMENT

If the scald or burn is:

- sustained by a baby or young child
- deep in character
- affects more than 10 per cent of the body surface (for example, a lower leg and foot or a whole arm)

the casualty should be taken to hospital without delay. No attempt should be made to remove burnt clothing. The burnt area should be covered with a clean sheet or pillow case. Nothing should be given by mouth (scc also page 76).

Smaller burns shoulds be treated by holding the area under a slowly running cold tap, or immersing in tepid water. This relieves the immediate pain. The burn should then be covered with a sterile dressing which is thick enough to exclude air. This may be held in place by a bandage or adhesive plaster. Any rings or bracelets should be removed before the area starts to swell. The patient will be upset by the incident; a cup of tea with a dose of aspirin or other pain-killer may be given to him and he should then rest quietly for a time.

## COT DEATHS

Many theories have been produced concerning the cause of death in babies who appear perfectly all right when put to sleep at night and then are found dead in the morning.

Not long ago this was thought to be due to suffocation, the child rolling on to its face and then unable to roll off the pillow or bedclothes. Obviously, soft pillows should never be used in cots or prams. Another dangerous habit which can cause suffocation is the practice of mother taking her crying baby to her own bed in the middle of the night. Both may drop off to sleep and the mother roll over on to the baby.

Sometimes vomitus from a baby forms a 'seal' between the nose, mouth and the bedclothes, and suffocation results. Another suffocation hazard of our time is the plastic bag or plastic sheeting used under cot sheets. Even those with punched holes should not be used where small children are around.

Reins or restrainers in perambulators are another potential danger. They should be secured firmly around the baby's body so that there is no danger of them working up to the baby's neck when he endeavours to get out of the pram.

## HEAT AND COLD

Measures should be taken to protect the eyes and skin from very strong sunlight and the extremities from excessive cold.

Babies must be kept warm and covered adequately. Elderly people should be encouraged to eat a well-balanced diet and take warm drinks and wear shawls. Ponchos, cardigans, mittens, bedsocks, or other extra coverings are advisable in very cold weather.

### Accidental hypothermia: indoors

Hypothermia produces various secondary pathological changes which have an important bearing on the clinical picture and on the patient's prognosis. (See also pages 156–9).

#### CLINICAL ASPECTS

Patients present with confusion, stupor, or even coma. The skin is pale, cold, dry, and corpse-like. A little oedema is present: this includes the face and at first glance suggests hypothyroidism (but the appearances are never so pronounced as in the hypothyroidism of myxoedema coma). Bradycardia is present sometimes with arrhythmia such as auricular fibrillation. Respiration is slowed and blood pressure lowered.

Hypothermia is considered to start at 32·2° C and from 26·7–32·2° C the outlook is quite good with proper treatment. Thereafter, the lower the temperature the more likely it is that the outcome will be fatal.

Exposure to cold is the overriding cause but endogenous factors are important. These include cerebrovascular accidents, conditions causing vascular collapse such as myocardial infarction, immobility, severe infection such as pneumonia, and drugs with hypothermic effects such as phenothiazines, barbiturates and alcohol.

#### TREATMENT

Active re-warming is known to be harmful. The usual explanation given is that it leads to dilation of cutaneous vessels, drawing blood away from more vital organs such as the heart and brain.

The casualty should be placed between blankets so that the body temperature recovers gradually. Subsequently, he should be nursed in a warm room at a temperature of approximately 32·2° C. Warm, sweet drinks may be given if the casualty is conscious.

## PREVENTION OF STREET ACCIDENTS TO CHILDREN

When advising parents on accident prevention in the home, it is necessary to remind them also of the potential hazards just outside the home and in travel to and from home.

Many street accidents are not the motorist's fault. Children should be taught kerb drill as soon as they can walk. Example is the best way of teaching and a habit formed in childhood can last a lifetime. While schools, television programmes and cinemas assist in teaching road safety, the ultimate responsibility must lie with parents. Children must learn that they must not run out into the road without looking; dash across the street after a ball or a thrown cap; run across to the ice cream vendor; or to pick up a conker. They should be taught never to hold on to a vehicle—even stationary ones can move off without warning.

They must know and observe notices in buses and underground trains and never stand on bus platforms. Instruction should be given also in the dangers of boarding or alighting from a moving train. Opening the door of a motor car or a railway carriage before it has stopped can cause an accident not only to oneself but also to others. Instruction on the safety code should be given to children: they must be taught never to hang on another vehicle whilst freewheeling on a bicycle or to overtake on the wrong side.

## FIRST AID KIT

In the average home, there is often little or nothing to use in an emergency. The bathroom cupboard frequently yields only some unidentifiable tablets, mouth wash, a pair of nail scissors and a bottle of aspirin. Cotton-wool and sticking plaster are sometimes in the house, but cannot always be found when needed.

It is sensible to gather together a few items which would be useful in an emergency and to keep these in a place where they are easily accessible to adults (Fig. 79). A metal or plastic box with a lid is required and should contain the following basic items:

Bandages: conforming and open weave, all sizes, one triangular.

Adhesive plasters and one roll of adhesive tape.

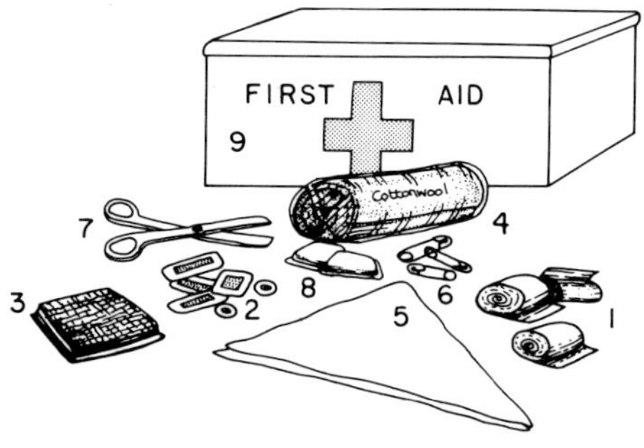


| | |
|---|---|
| 1 Bandages | 6 Pins |
| 2 Plasters and tape | 7 Scissors |
| 3 Gauze | 8 Dressings |
| 4 Cotton wool roll | 9 Tin or plastic box with lid |
| 5 Piece of white material | |

**Fig. 79** The basic requirements for a first aid box.

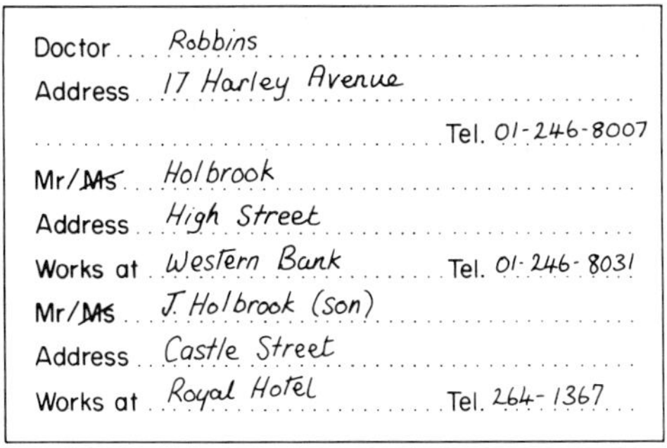


**Fig. 80** Card giving emergency addresses and telephone numbers.

Gauze.
Cotton-wool.
Pieces of old, clean white material, preferably cotton, for example, an old pillow-case.
Safety-pins.
Scissors.
Sterile prepared dressings.

(A more extensive list as recommended by the Voluntary Aid Societies is given in Appendix 1.)

Both in the first aid box and at a place near the telephone there should be a card, with the name, address and telephone numbers of doctor, hospital and all family members (Fig. 80). This will save valuable time if there is a major emergency.

CHAPTER 12

# Injuries in Sport

Many injuries sustained during sporting events can bc predicted. The type of injury will vary according to the sport concerned, but may be classified as direct or indirect.

Direct injuries are those which are caused by contact with an external object. A simple, but typical, example is the concussional head injury suffered by a boxer after receiving a blow on his chin, delivered by his opponent's gloved fist. Indirect injuries are those which are self-inflicted in the sense that they arise from repeated stress and overuse; a state which is frequently compounded by poor technique or by equipment. Together these factors can cause tissue damage or disruption. One example of this is 'tennis elbow' (or tendoperiostitis of the lateral epicondyle of the humerus), frequently encountered among tennis and squash players.

A majority of direct injuries sustained in sport are bruises, joint disruptions, fractures, lacerations and concussion. Indirect injuries usually involve the musculotendinous units and joints.

As always, the responsibility of the first aider is to assess the injury, arrive at a diagnosis and institute treatment to sustain life or to prevent deterioration of the victim's condition.

Two detailed surveys of the rate of injury in many of the popular participant sports in the United Kingdom are summarised in Table 3. In a sports injury report (Muckle & Shepherdson, 1975), with a rate for individuals per 100 participants, rugby football and skiing appear as the most dangerous sports—4·9 per 100. Closely following these are association football at 3·2, gymnastics at 2·9, and hockey at 2·7.

Injuries occurring during participation in a sport are also calculated by time—10 000 hours of play (Weightman & Browne, 1975)—and illustrated in Figure 81. Association football is shown to be the most

**Table 3** Sports injury rate per 100 participants

| | |
|---|---|
| Rugby | 4·9 |
| Skiing | 4·9 |
| Soccer | 3·2 |
| Gymnastics | 2·9 |
| Hockey | 2·7 |
| Judo | 2·1 |
| Rowing | 2·1 |
| Squash | 2·0 |
| Tennis | 2·0 |
| Boating | 1·7 |
| Basketball | 1·7 |

*Source:* Study by Muckle & Shepherdson published in Muckle D. S. (1978) *Injuries in Sport.* Bristol: John Wright.

dangerous—36·5 per 10 000 hours—with rugby football second at 30·5. Hockey, the third most dangerous, records a significant injury rate ranging between 12·5 for women and 10·3 for men.

The various sites of injury, related to each activity, are also identified in Figure 81. Injuries to the lower limb appear to predominate in the majority of sports, but there is a significant increase in the proportion of injuries sustained to the head and face among rugby, hockey and cricket players.

In England and Wales, fatalities occurring from sporting and leisure activities, excluding drowning, show rugby football to be the most dangerous of ball games. Motorcycling accounts for the highest rate of deaths in motor sports (see Table 4). Similar detailed figures do not exist for Scotland and Northern Ireland. It is, however, recognised that a significant number of deaths occur in the Scottish hills and, in 1979, 21 people died while hill walking.

## IMMEDIATE LIFE-THREATENING INJURIES

Respiratory and cardiac emergencies must be dealt with first as in any other context.

**Table 4** Sporting and leisure fatalities in England and Wales, 1977–78

| | 1977 Male | 1977 Female | 1978 Male | 1978 Female |
|---|---|---|---|---|
| Ball games | 9 | – | 10 | – |
| Football | 3 | – | 3 | – |
| Rugby | 3 | – | 4 | – |
| Cricket | 1 | – | 1 | – |
| Squash | 2 | – | 1 | – |
| Tennis | – | – | 1 | – |
| Athletic sports | 2 | – | 5 | – |
| Boxing | – | – | 1 | – |
| Cross-country | – | – | 1 | – |
| Jogging | – | – | 1 | – |
| Judo | 1 | – | – | – |
| Gymnastics | – | – | 2 | – |
| Unspecified | 1 | – | – | – |
| Motor sports | 17 | – | 17 | – |
| Karting | 2 | – | 3 | – |
| Car | 6 | – | – | – |
| Motor cycling | 9 | – | 14 | – |
| Water sports | 3 | – | – | – |
| Water skiing | 1 | – | – | – |
| Fishing | 1 | – | – | – |
| Unspecified | 1 | – | – | – |
| Air sports | 5 | 1 | 17 | – |
| Hang gliding | 3 | – | 6 | – |
| Gliding | 1 | 1 | 7 | – |
| Air display (plane) | 1 | – | – | – |
| Aircraft (unspecified) | – | – | 1 | – |
| Parachuting | – | – | 3 | – |
| Horse riding | 4 | 4 | 5 | 15 |
| Hunting | 1 | – | 1 | – |
| Gymkhana | – | 1 | – | – |
| Point-to-point | – | – | 1 | – |
| Unspecified | 3 | 3 | 3 | 15 |
| Mountaineering and climbing | 9 | – | 20 | 2 |
| Rock and cliff climbing | 7 | – | 7 | 1 |
| Fell walking | – | – | 1 | – |
| Unspecified | 2 | – | 12 | 1 |

*continued overleaf*

**Table 4** *continued*

| | 1977 Male | 1977 Female | 1978 Male | 1978 Female |
|---|---|---|---|---|
| Other sporting and leisure activities | 6 | 3 | 14 | – |
| Shooting | 1 | – | 1 | – |
| Cycling | – | – | 1 | – |
| Skateboarding | 1 | – | 4 | – |
| Sledging | 1 | – | 1 | – |
| Flying model aircraft | 1 | – | – | – |
| Children's playground | 1 | 1 | – | – |
| Fairground | 1 | 2 | 5 | – |
| Billiards | – | – | 1 | – |
| Navigation competition | – | – | 1 | – |
| Spectators | 2 | – | 2 | – |
| Football | – | – | 1 | – |
| Motor racing | 2 | – | 1 | – |

The figures exclude: drowning and deaths in which the victims' activities are considered part of their occupation.
*Source:* Office of Population Censuses and Surveys.

## COMA

A patient may lose consciousness following airway obstruction, cardiac arrest or shock but on the sports field it is likely to be the result of a head injury. Treatment is the same in all sitings.

## CERVICAL SPINE INJURY

Fracture dislocation of the cervical spine is fortunately rare in sport but the possibility must always be borne in mind. It may be caused by a heavy fall; tackling or collapse of the scrum in rugby football or a whiplash injury sustained in diving.

## EXTERNAL HAEMORRHAGE

Rapid external haemorrhage from a major vessel can lead to shock and death. This may happen in motor-racing.

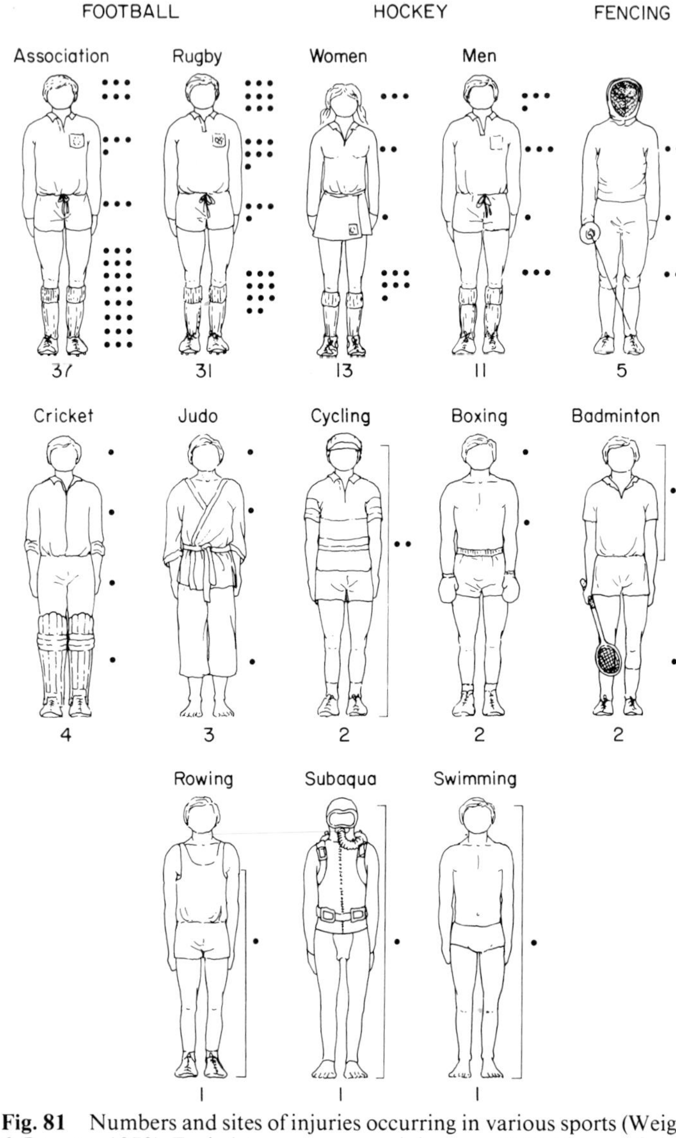


**Fig. 81** Numbers and sites of injuries occurring in various sports (Weightman & Browne, 1979). Each dot represents one injury per 10 000 hours of play.

## INTERNAL INJURIES

Internal injuries to the chest and abdomen following a direct blow can cause fractured ribs (including a flail chest), pneumothorax, internal haemorrhage into either the chest or the abdomen or cardiac injury or arrest. They may occur during a fall from a horse, or during football or rugby matches and the like.

The patient will have been winded. Early recovery from winding is best achieved by allowing the patient time to rest. Other signs and symptoms will vary according to the injury sustained. Detailed examination away from the field of play may be needed before an accurate diagnosis can be made.

## COMMON DIRECT INJURIES

The majority of injuries sustained during sporting activities are due to direct violence following collision with: an opponent, often at speed; an instrument or equipment used in the sport; the ground; or the walls of a court (for example, in squash).

### Bruises; haematomata; torn muscles

Bruises are caused by bleeding into the tissues following a direct blow. The bleeding may be subcutaneous or it may be into the muscle compartments. If the injury causes rupture of the muscle bundles, the bleeding disperses readily and is classified as an intramuscular haematoma. With intermuscular bleeding, the bruising cannot readily disperse as it is confined within the muscle bundles.

A group of muscle fibres within a major muscle may rupture during violent activity and this will also cause bleeding and bruising within the muscle bundles.

#### CAUSES

A direct blow or a spontaneous muscle rupture during strenuous activity.

#### SIGNS AND SYMPTOMS

Pain, swelling, and impaired function.

TREATMENT

Immediate treatment to stop further bleeding into the tissue is the primary objective. The 4 steps to be taken are sometimes more easily remembered by the acronym RICE:

REST Stop the activity to reduce the overall circulation and prevent further tissue disruption.

ICE The application of ice to the injured part for 2 minutes will cool the injured tissues without causing a rebound injury to local blood flow. Ice will also relieve pain and spasm, but the skin *must* be protected from ice-burning by first applying a thin coat of petroleum jelly.

COMPRESSION A circumferential compression bandage should be applied to achieve further reduction of bleeding into the tissues.

ELEVATION Elevation of the injured part will also reduce blood flow to the injured part.

The immediate adoption of the RICE measures will facilitate early recovery. Supplemented by physiotherapy, rehabilitation (which should start approximately 36 to 48 hours after injury, when all danger of further bleeding into the tissues has been minimised) will usually be rapid.

## Joint disruptions

Ligaments, capsule, synovium or joint surfaces are frequently damaged in sport. The joints most commonly involved are the knee, ankle and shoulder girdle. Accurate diagnosis immediately after injury can be extremely difficult, especially when dealing with the knee joint, because of the close anatomical relationships between the joint structures. The knee can also suffer damage to the menisci, when the femur crushes the cartilage against the tibia.

CAUSE

Injuries to the knee and ankle occur when the momentum of the body is transferred through the joint and the foot remains firmly on the ground. The shoulder girdle is injured by transmitted forces following a fall on the outstretched upper limb or on the lateral aspect of the shoulder.

TREATMENT

The immediate first aid care of such injuries follows the principles outlined previously, namely: Rest, Ice, Compression, and Elevation. Knees and ankles often benefit also from early temporary immobilisation by splints. Injuries to the shoulder girdle are better supported by a triangular sling bandage.

If an effusion develops rapidly in the knee joint, immediately after injury, or if the knee locks, the patient must be transferred to hospital for further assessment.

Minor dislocations of the interdigital joints or of the glenohumeral shoulder 'joint' can be reduced immediately after injury if someone present is competent in the appropriate technical skill. Major dislocations of large joints such as the elbow, knee or ankle can cause significant ischaemic damage to the adjacent structures because of the degree of deformity present, for example skin necrosis, vessel or nerve damage. The patient should be transferred to hospital as quickly as possible.

## Fractures

Assessment of the fractures sustained in sport is similar to that described in Chapter 5. Many fractures will be relatively minor such as digits, nasal bones and the like. Fractures of the long bone or ribs can occur and may be associated with internal injuries.

CAUSE

Heavy falls, often as a result of a collision between opponents.

SIGNS AND SYMPTOMS

Pain, swelling, deformity, crepitus, abnormal movement and loss of function are the cardinal signs of a fracture. It is important to identify whether there is also a wound in the skin, as such a communication between the skin and the fracture site greatly increases the liability to infection.

TREATMENT

Basic aims of treatment are to ensure that any associated wound is protected from contamination and that the fracture site is immobilised.

The immobilisation of both minor and major fractures is the most effective technique to reduce blood loss. This can initially be achieved by the first-aider supporting the fracture site with her or his hands. But as soon as possible, bandaging and a triangular sling (for upper limbs) and padded wooden or air splints (for lower limbs) should be applied. The injury must also be assessed for possible internal complicating injuries, for example compression of the brachial artery. This may occur when there is a supracondylar fracture at the elbow joint.

Bleeding into minor fracture sites can also be minimised by the measures outlined earlier, using Ice, Compression bandaging, and Elevation.

## Lacerations

Lacerations commonly occur in sport, and all participants should be fully protected against tetanus.

### CAUSES

Linear lacerations commonly follow a clash of heads (such as during a rugby scrum) where the skin splits over a bony prominence, such as the eyebrow. Bursting stellate lacerations occur as a result of injury from studs of an opponent's boots in soccer. These are often contaminated with dirt. Puncture wounds are sometimes caused by running spikes. Abrasions from a fall can be very painful and also slow to heal. Differentiation should be based on a history of the incident and the appearance of the wound.

### TREATMENT

Linear lacerations are best treated by cleaning with an antiseptic such as Iodophor solution and covering with a padded sterile compression bandage. The player can frequently return to his sport immediately.

Adhesive tape sutures may be used but they often fail to stick on to a perspiring forehead! If appropriate facilities are available, the wound may be sutured.

Stellate lacerations, which are frequently contaminated, must be cleaned thoroughly and dressed. Transfer to a facility where appropriate exploration and suturing can be undertaken under anaesthesia should be arranged.

Puncture wounds should be cleansed thoroughly and the wound insufflated with Iodophor powder prior to the application of a dressing.

Abrasions are best cleaned with running, soapy water and left exposed to allow the surface to dry. If for some reason this is not possible, a non-adherent dressing should be applied.

## Concussion

Concussion follows a temporary disturbance of normal brain function when there is a partial or complete brief loss of consciousness associated with a period of amnesia. The latter may be very brief.

Concussion should *never* be treated as a minor event nor regarded lightly. First, repeated concussional episodes can lead to permanent brain damage. This has been clearly recognised by those authorities who regulate boxing. A boxer who has been concussed in a bout is not allowed to train or box for at least 3 weeks and then only if passed fit by a doctor. This precaution aims to minimise the prospect of developing the 'punch drunk syndrome' in later life.

The second risk is the possibility of a transient concussion being associated with a slow haemorrhage which progressively compresses the brain. In these circumstances the concussed player has a lucid interval, which may last several hours, followed by gradual deterioration of his or her conscious level to coma and if untreated to death. The incidence of concussion and coma can be significantly reduced by participants using properly fitted mouth guards. Preferably this use should be supervised by the player's own dentist.

### CAUSE

A direct blow to the jaw or skull.

### SIGNS AND SYMPTOMS

Mild confusion, a transient amnesia, visual disturbance, headaches or nausea. Irritability can also be a feature. A change of conscious level is a sign of progressive deterioration.

### TREATMENT

The patient must rest quietly and *not* be left alone. Alcohol or analgesics should not be given.

Medical assessment and a period of observation, preferably in a hospital, are essential.

## COMMON INDIRECT AND OVERUSE INJURIES

### Musculotendinous rupture

Spontaneous rupture of the musculotendinous junction can occur in the hamstring and calf muscles, during sprinting. It can also occur in the muscles of the upper limb in throwing events such as cricket and throwing the discus. It can be a recurring problem, particularly among stocky individuals.

#### CAUSE

Inadequate warm-up before beginning strenuous activity, aggravated by fatigue.

#### SIGNS AND SYMPTOMS

Loss of normal function, local tenderness, a boggy swelling and adjacent muscle spasm which can prevent active contraction of the muscle group or passive stretching.

#### TREATMENT

Immediate treatment follows the RICE measures (Rest, Ice, Compression and Elevation).

Definitive care will be designed to maintain the length of the musculotendinous unit.

Thereafter, the coach will design a modified rehabilitation programme to ensure full recovery.

### Achilles peritendonitis

Achilles peritendonitis can be either focal degeneration within the Achilles tendon or inflammation of the tendon sheath. The latter is a chronic overuse condition frequently exacerbated by the stress of competing in a specific event. Differential diagnosis can be extremely difficult.

#### CAUSE

The condition develops as a result of a chronic overuse injury. It is commonly found in individuals whose training schedules have involved considerable time spent running on hard surfaces, particularly at the beginning of a training schedule. The most common causative factor is the use of poor quality running shoes. It is particularly encountered in women athletes, who wear shoes with a high or medium heel during most of their daily activities and then use flat-heeled or spiked running shoes for training purposes.

SIGNS AND SYMPTOMS

Loss of function and a tender oedematous swelling around the Achilles tendon.

TREATMENT

The immediate treatment is based on minimising the inflammatory response and this is best achieved by the RICE technique described to control blood loss into the tissues.

Later, a cushioned heel-raise should be inserted in the player's normal shoe, and the female athlete should be warned against wearing high heels, and the male, against wearing stacked-heeled shoes or boots.

Once again, definitive care can be a prolonged exercise requiring the skills of physiotherapist, doctor and coach.

## Chondromalacia patellae

The unusual condition of chondromalacia patellae is due to flaking of cartilage on the undersurface of a patella.

CAUSE

The cause is not known but it is thought to be caused by repeated episodes of minor jarring trauma and some weakness of the vastus medialis muscle in the quadriceps muscle group.

SIGNS AND SYMPTOMS

Pain deep to the patella and, on palpation, of its undersurface. A small effusion may be present in the knee joint. Some loss of muscle bulk in the thigh will be apparent.

TREATMENT

Immediate care for this condition is based on minimising the effusion. A compression bandage, for example a double layer of tubigrip (Seton) should be applied, reinforced by a horseshoe made of non-compressible felt (Fig. 82).

Thereafter, continued care will involve specialist advice.

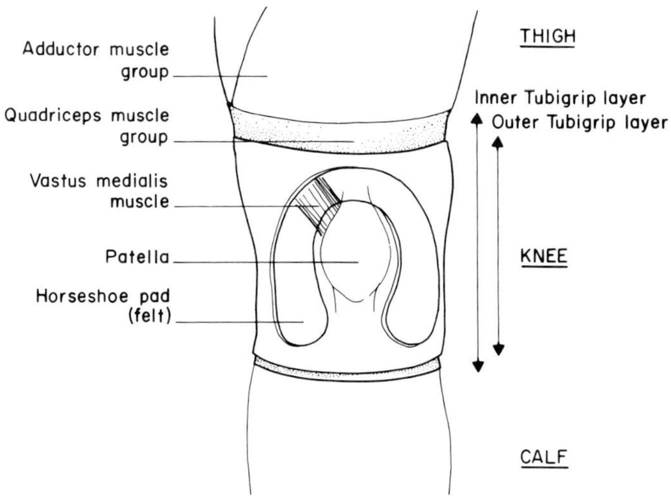


**Fig. 82** Application of a compression bandage and horseshoe pad to the knee joint.

## Tibial compartment compression syndromes

A range of conditions in middle- and long-distance runners are described under the general term of *Shin splints.* The term covers:

a stress fracture of the tibia
tendoperiostitis of the tibial muscle attachments to the shin
tibial muscle-compartment compression

Tibial compartment compression can cause muscle infarction and result in permanent loss of function it if is not recognised and treated rapidly. It can effect either the tibialis anterior or tibialis posterior muscles.

CAUSE
Unknown, but believed to be a result of muscle engorgement and oedema in the rigid compartment bounded by the tibia, the interosseus membrane and the deep fascia.

SIGNS AND SYMPTOMS
Loss of function with pain and tenderness over the length of the muscle involved. Passive stretching of the muscle causes severe pain.

TREATMENT
The leg should be elevated and ice applied locally. After a short period, a compression bandage may be applied. Light massage of the involved muscle compartment can help. If rapid relief of the symptoms is not achieved, the patient must be immediately transferred to hospital. It may be necessary to decompress the compartment surgically to prevent infarction and subsequent fibrosis.

## ILLNESSES PRECIPITATED BY SPORT

Travelling parties are commonly subject to upper respiratory tract infections and sport teams are no exception. These infections are caused by air-conditioning, central heating, the variations in atmospheric pressure when flying and the enforced proximity of a large group of travellers.

TREATMENT
It is best to limit treatment to simple antipyrexial agents such as aspirin, and a decongestant inhalation of steam and Friar's balsam.

Traveller's diarrhoea, known by many colourful names such as Montezuma's revenge, is caused by a change of diet and water and is frequently aggravated by alcohol cooled with contaminated ice cubes. The use of prophylactic antibiotics in an attempt to maintain a sterile gastrointestinal tract is not recommended. The travelling party should be advised against taking risky water and items of food, for example uncooked meat, unwashed fruit and salad vegetables, ice cream. If diarrhoea does develop, it should be treated by simple agents such as codeine phosphate. Persistent diarrhoea or the passage of blood with mucus requires medical attention.

In the presence of one of these systemic febrile illnesses, relatively minor sporting activities may precipitate an emergency condition.

## Cardiovascular disease

CAUSES

Viral myocarditis.
Congenital heart disease.
Cardiomyopathy.

The conditions listed are invariably asymptomatic until the time of collapse. Sudden death can occur in the middle-aged athlete as a result of coronary artery disease, leading to myocardial infarction. Such circumstances are also reported in the 30- to 40-year age group. In many instances the athletes dying in these circumstances have tended to ignore apparently trivial symptoms such as undue fatigue, minor exertional chest pain, or palpitations.

Collapse and death following rupture of a subarachnoid 'berry' aneurysm or a stroke can also occur in athletes of a wide age-range. The underlying pathology in these circumstances will have invariably been silent.

SIGNS AND SYMPTOMS

The diagnosis of cardiac arrest is based on the absence of pulsation at the carotid or femoral vessels, the cessation of respiratory effort, and dilating pupils.

TREATMENT

External cardiac massage in conjunction with mouth-to-mouth artificial respiration must be instituted immediately (see Chap. 2).

## Haematuria

CAUSE

The presence of blood in the urine of an athlete is most often the result of a direct blow. Haematuria, however, has been frequently identified in middle- to long-distance runners and in long-distance walkers. The causes remain uncertain but haemolysis of red cells, jarring of the kidneys and dehydration have been blamed.

TREATMENT

Haematuria normally resolves with rest. To eliminate any other possible cause of haematuria, such as a congenital abnormality of the urinary tract, the sportsman or woman should be told to see his own doctor for a thorough examination.

## ENVIRONMENTAL ILLNESSES

Environmental illnesses incorporate heat exhaustion, dehydration, salt depletion and hypothermia.

### Heat exhaustion/dehydration/salt depletion

CAUSE

A complex disturbance of the normal body homeostasis can result from repeated or prolonged exercise in a hot and humid environment. This is often aggravated by the wearing of clothing which prevents adequate skin cooling. The core temperature of the body rises in conjunction with sweat loss, and subsequent dehydration and electrolyte imbalance occurs.

SIGNS AND SYMPTOMS

The patient will become confused, suffer from cramps and will eventually collapse.

TREATMENT

Immediate treatment should be aimed at cooling the body surface by fanning a cool breeze over the exposed skin.

Gradual oral rehydration with appropriate glucose and salt supplements should also be initiated.

### Hypothermia

Hypothermia, which can lead to collapse and even death, is caused by the rapid loss of heat from the body core (see pages 155–7 also). This commonly occurs as a result of a combination of wet, cold environmental circumstances aggravated by the wind. These conditions are frequently encountered by hill-walkers, mountaineers and water-sports participants. In seas around northern Britain, death from hypothermia can occur in under 15 minutes, and even more rapidly if heat is wasted in unproductive attempts at swimming.

Prevention of hypothermia by careful planning of any expedition, wearing appropriate insulated clothing, avoiding exhaustion and ensuring a diet high in carbohydrates will minimise the incidence of the condition.

### SIGNS AND SYMPTOMS

Patients may only initially show features of clumsiness and irrational behaviour but these can rapidly progress to total collapse.

### TREATMENT

Treatment varies with the circumstances, but as soon as the condition is suspected there is no time for delay. Any patient suffering from hypothermia must be sheltered from further heat loss by protection from the wind. If at all possible, he or she should be changed into dry clothing and wrapped in an insulated sleeping bag or in a hypothermia bag. A warm, dry companion sharing the sleeping bag or hypothermia bag will speed the warming process.

Wherever possible, further active warming should be instituted by the provision of warm, sweetened drinks and carbohydrate supplements. Alcohol *should not* be given, as this tends to delay the raising of the patient's core temperature.

CHAPTER 13

# Moving and Carrying Injured Persons

## TRANSPORT OF CASUALTIES

Before moving a casualty, unless life is endangered by fire, falling masonry, poisonous atmosphere, or other perilous conditions, it is important to carry out a quick but systematic examination and provide support or transport or both as appropriate.

A sick or injured person may be removed to shelter by the following methods:

- support by a single helper
- handseats and chair-carry
- blanket lift
- stretcher
- wheeled transport
- air or sea transport.

The method to be adopted (and it may be necessary to use more than one) will depend upon:

- the nature and severity of the injury
- the number of helpers and the facilities available
- the distance to shelter or hospital or both
- the nature of the route to be travelled.

The aim should be to see that the casualty reaches his or her destination without the condition becoming worse. The following three principles must be regularly kept in mind.

**1** The position assumed by the casualty, or in which he or she has been placed, must not be altered unnecessarily.

**2** Throughout transport, a careful watch must be kept on:

- the general condition of the casualty
- the maintenance of an open airway

the control of bleeding

the continuous immobilisation of fractures and large wounds

**3** The transport must be safe and steady.

## METHODS OF CARRYING

If help is available, do not attempt to move a seriously ill or injured casualty on your own.

### Cradle

The cradle is for casualities of light weight or children. Lift the casualty by passing one of your arms well beneath the two knees, and the other round the neck.

### Human crutch

Standing at the casualty's injured side, except where there is injury to an upper limb, assist the casualty by putting your arm round the waist, grasping his or her clothing at the hip, and placing the casualty's arm round your neck, holding his or her hand with your free hand (Fig. 83a).

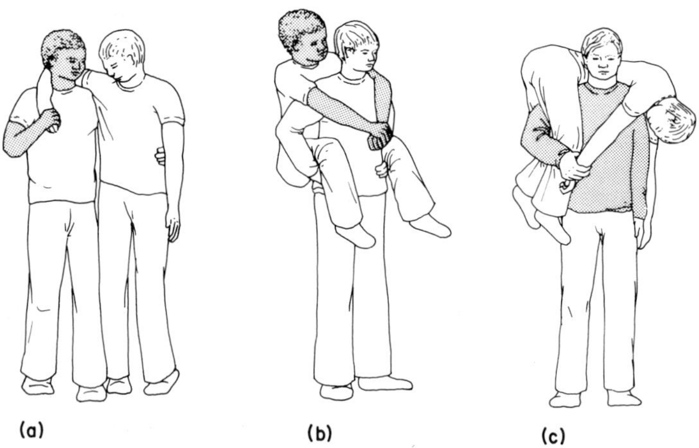


**Fig. 83** Transport of a casualty by one person: (a) human crutch, (b) pick-a-back and (c) fireman's lift and carry.

If the upper limbs are uninjured and the casualty's other hand is free, he or she may gain additional help from a staff or walking stick.

**Pick-a-back**

If the casualty is conscious and able to hold on, he or she may be carried in the ordinary pick-a-back fashion (Fig. 83b).

**Fireman's lift and carry**

Help the casualty to rise to the upright position. Grasp his or her right wrist with your left hand. Bend your head down under the casualty's extended right arm so that your right shoulder is level with the lower part of his or her abdomen, and place your right arm between or round the legs. Taking the weight on your right shoulder, rise to the erect position. Pull the casualty across both shoulders and transfer his or her right wrist to your right hand, so leaving your left hand free (Fig. 83c).

**By two or more helpers**

*Four-handed seat*

The four-handed seat is used when the casualty can assist by using one or both arms.

Two helpers face each other behind the casualty and grasp their left wrists with their right hands and each other's right wrists with their left hands and stoop down (Fig. 84a).

The casualty is instructed to place one arm around the neck of each helper to raise himself or herself to sit on their hands for steadying during transport (Fig. 84b).

The helpers rise together and step off with outside feet and walk with ordinary paces forward.

*Two-handed seat*

The two-handed seat is mostly used to carry a casualty who is unable to assist by using his or her arms.

Two helpers face each other and stoop, one on each side of the casualty. Each helper passes her or his forearm nearest the casualty's body under the back, just below the shoulders and, if possible, takes hold of clothing (Fig. 85a). They raise the casualty's back slightly and then pass their other forearms under the middle of the casualty's

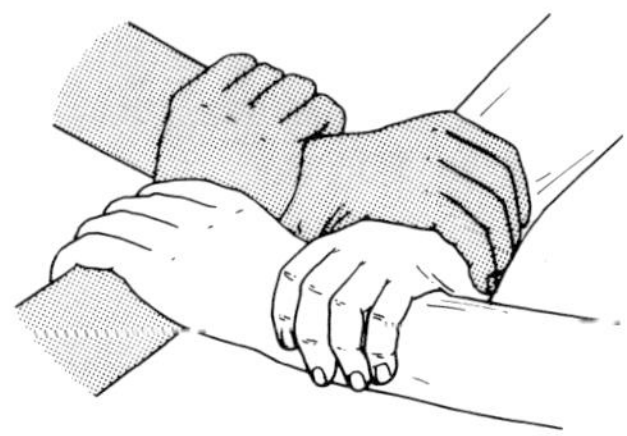
(a)

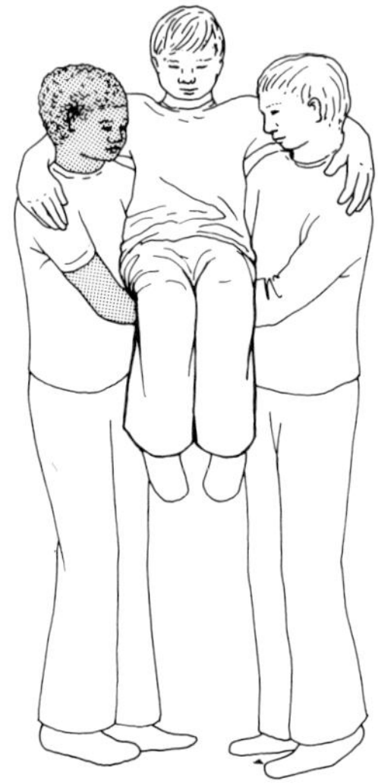
(b)

**Fig. 84** Four-handed seat showing (a) the wrist grasp and (b) the carry.

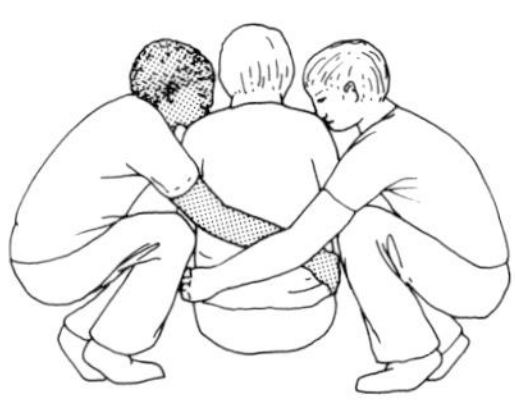
(a)

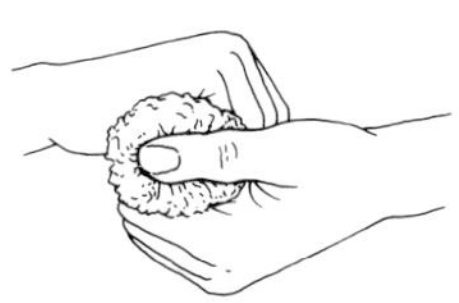
(b)

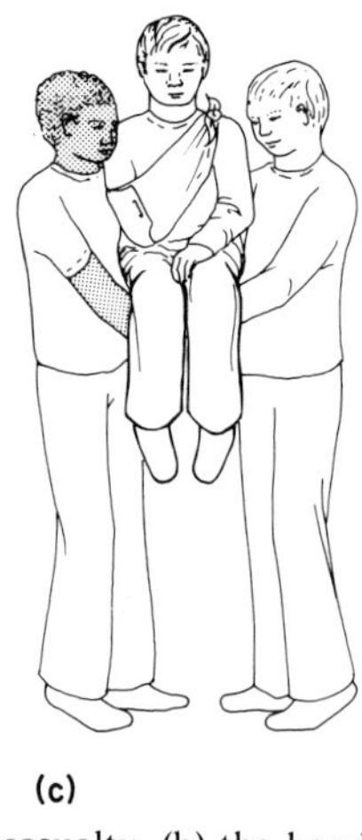
(c)

**Fig. 85** Two-handed seat showing (a) supporting the casualty, (b) the hand clasp and (c) the carry.

thighs and clasp their hands (Fig. 85b), the helper on the left of the casualty with palm upwards and holding a folded handkerchief to prevent hurting by the fingernails; the helper on the right of the casualty with palms downwards (hook-grip).

The helpers rise together and step off with outside feet (Fig. 85c). In all cases of carrying by hand seats, the crossover step and not side paces will be used.

*Kitchen chair method*

When a casualty, conscious and without serious injuries is to be moved up or down stairs or along passageways, an ordinary kitchen-type chair can be used (Fig. 86). The way should first of all be cleared of furniture or other obstruction.

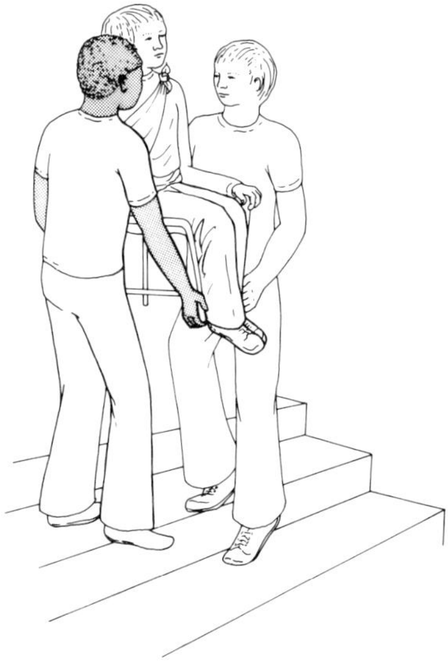

**Fig. 86** The kitchen chair method.

The casualty should be seated on the chair and supported by helpers, front and rear. The chair and the casualty are then slowly tilted backwards to an angle of 30° to the horizontal and lifted.

One helper should support the back of the chair and the casualty; the other, facing the casualty, should hold the chair by the front legs and move carefully backwards down the stairs.

If the stairs or passageway are wide enough, the helpers can stand at the sides of the chair, each supporting a back and front leg of the chair.

## PREPARING AND BLANKETING A STRETCHER

Two helpers open and secure the stretcher, ensuring that the traverses are fully opened. The stretcher is then tested by one person lying on it and the two ends of the stretcher raised off the ground in turn, to ensure the bed will take the weight of the casualty. Then the stretcher is blanketed according to the number of blankets available.

**With one blanket**

Place the blanket diagonally over the stretcher (Fig. 87).

After placing the the casualty on the stretcher:

carry the point of the blanket round the neck and on to the chest

the point of the blanket at the foot is brought up over the casualty's feet and a small fold tucked between the ankles to prevent rubbing

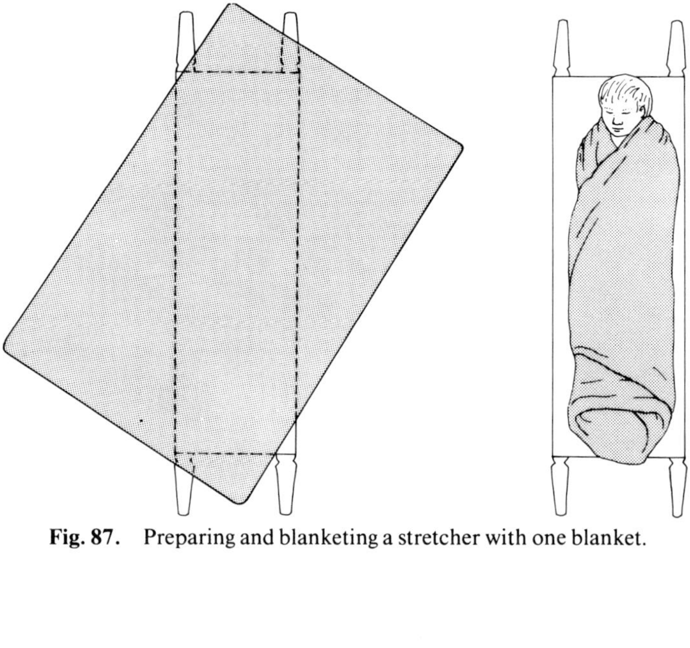

**Fig. 87.** Preparing and blanketing a stretcher with one blanket.

the right side of the blanket is carried over the casualty and tucked in

the left side of the blanket is brought over and tucked in

**With two blankets**

Place the first blanket lengthwise across the stretcher with one edge covering half the handles at the head, and slightly more to one side of the stretcher than the other.

Fold the second blanket lengthwise into three and place on the stretcher with the upper edge about 45 cm below the upper edge of the first blanket. Open out the folds at the lower end for about 60 cm (Fig. 88a).

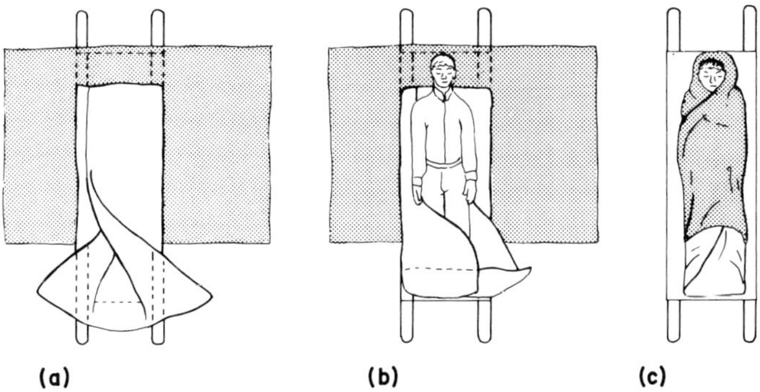


**Fig. 88** Preparing and blanketing a stretcher with two blankets: (a) position of each blanket and (b) casualty on the stretcher and (c) wrapping the casualty in the blankets.

After placing the casualty on the stretcher:

the foot of the second blanket is brought over the casualty's feet and a small fold tucked between the ankles to prevent rubbing

the open folds of the blanket are then brought over the legs and feet and tucked in (Fig. 88b)

the upper corners of the first blanket are turned in and the shorter side brought over the casualty and tucked in

the longer side of the blanket is then brought over and tucked in (Fig. 88c)

## LOADING A STRETCHER

**Four bearers**

A squad of four, numbered 1 to 4 are required. All orders are given by No. 1.

*Casualty lying on a blanket*

The bearers place themselves on each side of the casualty. Nos. 1 and 2 at the feet and Nos. 3 and 4 at the head.

The edges of the blanket are rolled against the side of the casualty and each bearer firmly grasps the rolled edges with hands about 6 inches apart. At the command of No. 1, the casualty is carefully and evenly lifted and unless a fifth person is available to slide the stretcher under the casualty, the four bearers will move with short even sidesteps until the casualty is directly over the canvas bed. He or she is then gently lowered on to it (Fig. 89c).

*Casualty not lying on a blanket but one is available*

The casualty should be placed on the blanket and then lifted on to the stretcher as described above (Fig. 89a, b and c).

*Casualty not lying on a blanket and none is available*

When the casualty is ready for loading on to the stretcher, Nos. 2, 3 and 4 will place themselves on the left of the casualty:

No. 2 facing the knees.
No. 3 facing the hips.
No. 4 facing the shoulders.

No. 1 will stand on the right of the casualty facing No. 3 (Fig. 90a).

All will go down on their left knees and place their forearms beneath the casualty, paying particular attention to the site of the injury. Using the hook-grip, No. 1 joins the left hand with the left hand of No. 4 and the right hand with the right hand of No. 3. No. 4 supports the head and shoulders, No. 2 the lower limbs.

When No. 1 gives the order: Lift, and casualty must be lifted gently, slowly, and evenly and placed on the knees of Nos. 2, 3 and 4 (Fig. 90b). No. 1 will disengage, get the prepared stretcher and place it under the casualty, so that when he or she is lowered on to it, the head will just be clear of the traverse at the top and will rest on the pillow. No. 1 will

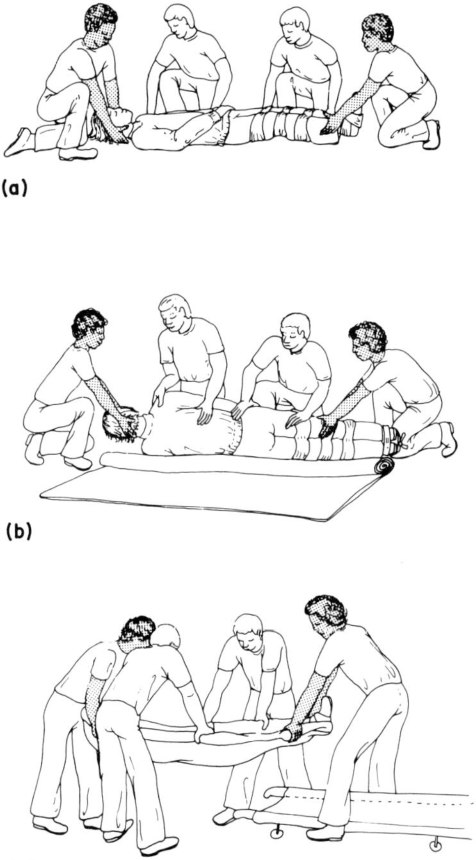

(a)

(b)

(c)

**Fig. 89** The blanket lift showing (a) preparation, (b) rolling the casualty onto the blanket and (c) lifting the casualty.

then resume her or his position and rejoin hands with bearers Nos. 4 and 2.

When No. 1 gives the order: Lower, the casualty will be raised slightly from the knees of the bearers, and then lowered gently, slowly, and evenly on to the stretcher bed (Fig. 90c). The bearers then rise and turn to face the foot of the stretcher. If lifting the casualty from the right side, bearers go down on their right knees.

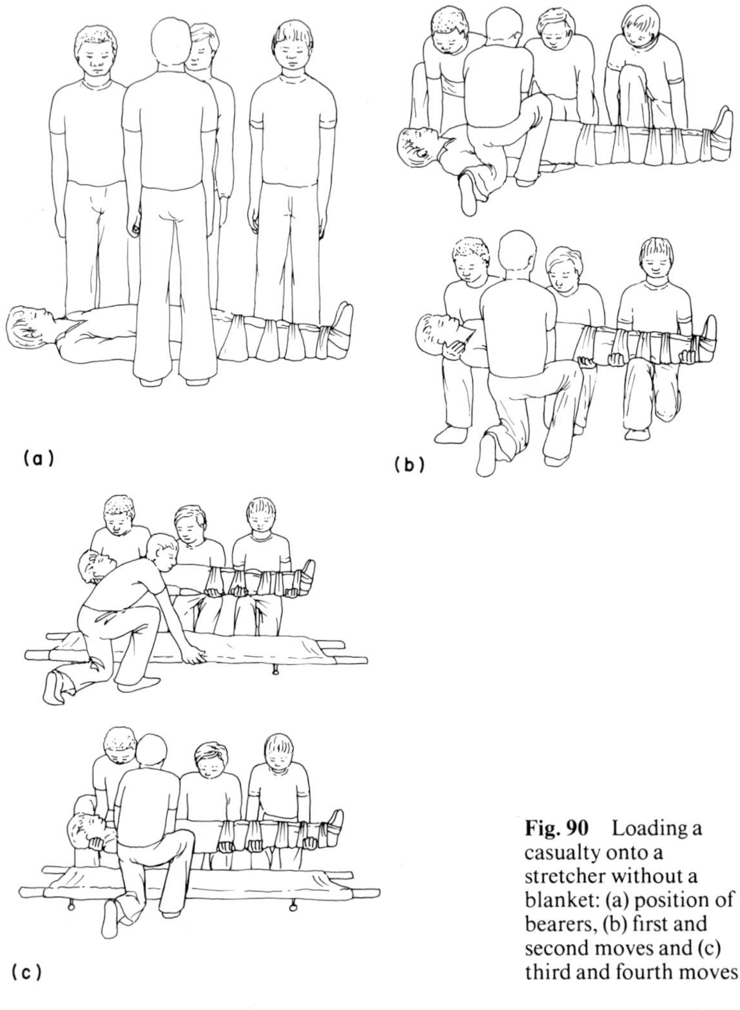


**Fig. 90** Loading a casualty onto a stretcher without a blanket: (a) position of bearers, (b) first and second moves and (c) third and fourth moves.

### Three bearers

When only three bearers are available, the stretcher will be placed at the casualty's head in line with his body. No. 1 will kneel on the left knee on the injured side opposite the casualty's knees, and passes the hands under the casualty's legs; Nos. 2 and 3 kneel on their left knees on opposite sides of the casualty; they pass their hands under his or her shoulders and hips and lock their fingers in the hook-grip (Fig. 91a). On the command: Lift, the bearers will rise to the erect position and, moving by side paces, carrying the casualty head first over the foot of the stretcher, the horizonal position of the body being maintained throughout the movement (Fig. 91b). The casualty is then lowered carefully on to the stretcher.

When unloading, the casualty will be uplifted and carried head foremost over the head of the stretcher.

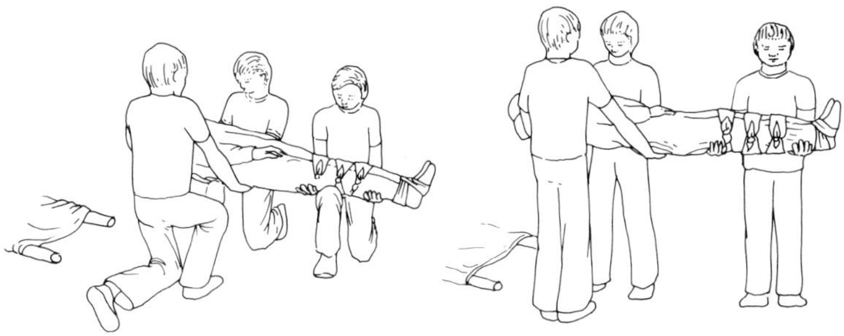

(a) (b)

**Fig. 91** The three-bearer lift: (a) position of kneeling bearers and (b) bearers standing up with the casualty in a horizontal position.

**Two bearers**

For use in mines and cuttings where space is limited.

The stretcher will be placed at the casualty's head in line with the body. Both bearers will stand astride the casualty, with No. 2 at the head, placing the forearms under the casualty's shoulders, No. 1 about the knees, placing the left hand beneath the casualty's thighs and the right below the knees. When both are ready, No. 1 will give the command: Lift. When the command Advance is given, both will step off together with the left foot taking short, even paces and stooping so that the body of the casualty is not far from the ground (Fig. 92a). They will advance until the casualty is over the stretcher, when No. 1 gives the order: Halt. Lower. The casualty is lowered gently on to the

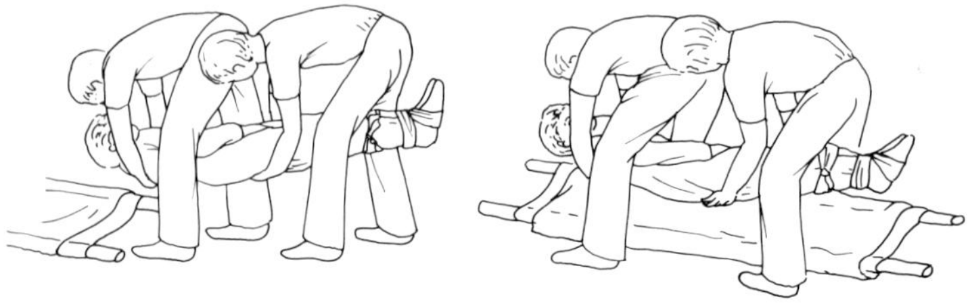

(a) (b)

**Fig. 92** The two-bearer lift: (a) carrying the casualty and (b) lowering the casualty onto the stretcher.

stretcher (Fig. 92b). Both bearers then take up position on the left of the stretcher ready for lifting, No. 2 at the head and No. 1 at the foot.

## CARRYING A STRETCHER

No. 1 will decide whether the stretcher is to be carried by two or four bearers. When the casualty has been placed on the stretcher, the bearers will take up their positions alongside the stretcher:

No. 1 at the foot of the stretcher on the right.
No. 2 at the foot of the stretcher on the left.
No. 3 at the head of the stretcher on the right.
No. 4 at the head of the stretcher on the left.

### By four bearers

On the command: Hand carriage by four bearers, all four bearers will stoop together and grasp the handles with their inner hands. On the command Lift, the bearers will rise together, holding the stretcher at the full extent of their arms. At the command: Advance, all bearers step off with the inner foot, keeping their knees slightly bent and walking with a relaxed gait (Fig. 93).

On the command: Lower stretcher, the four bearers will stoop, gently lower the stretcher to the ground and then rise together.

### By two bearers

On the command Hand carriage by two bearers, Nos. 2 and 4 will then take side paces over the handles of the stretcher, and if slings are to be

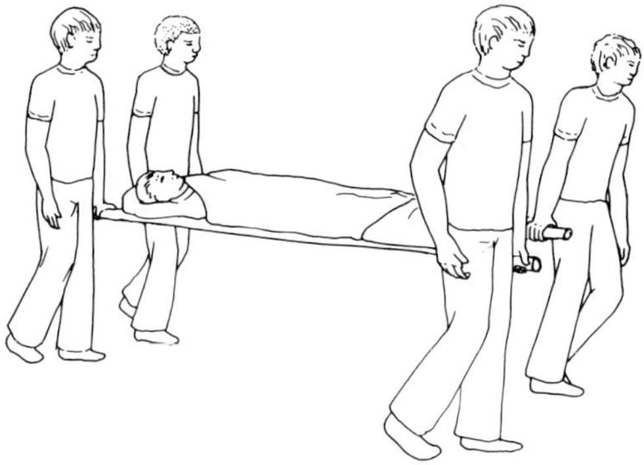

**Fig. 93** Carrying a stretcher with four bearers.

used, they will place them over their shoulders and on the handles of the stretcher. On the command Lift, the two bearers will rise together keeping the stretcher level. Nos. 1 and 3 will turn inwards to assist. No. 1 particularly can help to prevent the casualty's feet catching the buttocks of No. 2.

On the command: Adjust slings, Nos. 1 and 3 turn to the left and adjust the slings of Nos. 2 and 4 respectively.

On the command: Advance, Nos. 1, 2 and 3 will step off with their left feet and No. 4 with the right. Bearers must keep their knees slightly bent and walk with a relaxed gait (Fig. 94).

On the command: Lower stretcher, Nos. 2 and 4 stoop slowly, and evenly and gently lower the stretcher to the ground, then rise together.

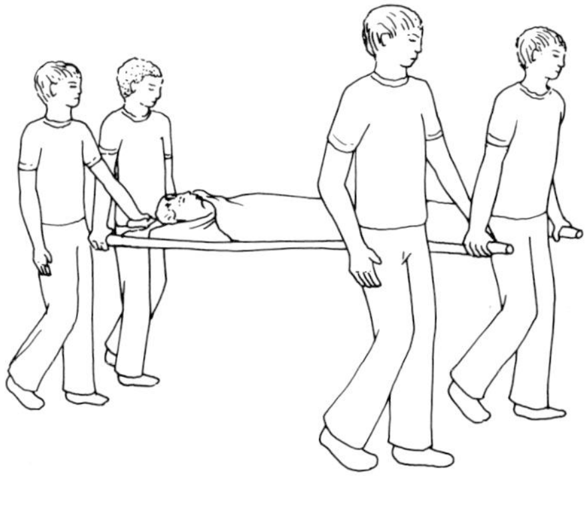

**Fig. 94** Carrying a stretcher with two bearers.

If slings are used, Nos. 2 and 4 will remove them and after lowering the stretcher will step over the handles and take up their former positions, placing the loops of the folded slings over the near handles and the ends over the other handles.

## UNLOADING A STRETCHER

On the command: Unload stretcher, the bearers will adopt a similar procedure to that carried out in loading the stretcher.

If the casualty is lying on a blanket, the blanket lift should be used. Where there is no blanket, after the casualty has been lifted to the bearers' knees, No. 1 will remove the stretcher and place it beyond the casualty's feet (Fig. 95).

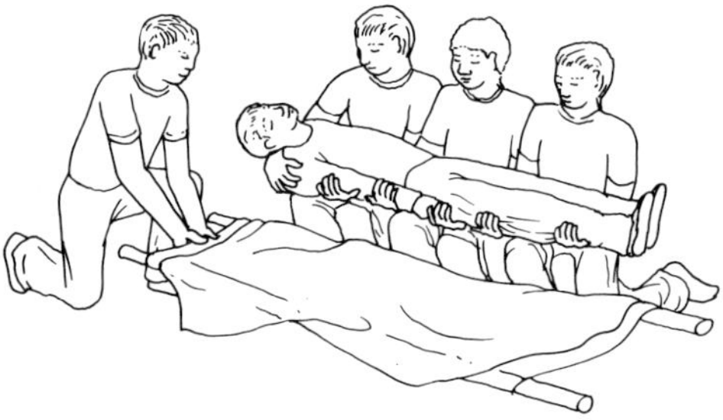

**Fig. 95** Unloading a stretcher.

## TO CLOSE A STRETCHER

Nos. 2 and 4 unlock the traverses and then push the poles together, fold the canvas on itself and buckle the straps tightly round the stretcher behind the traverses. When slings are used, they are placed along the canvas and the straps buckled round the stretcher behind the traverses. If a telescopic-handled type stretcher is used, the handles must be pushed home.

## IMPROVISED STRETCHERS

Stretchers may be improvised in one of the following ways:

**1** Turn the sleeves of two or three coats inside out; pass two strong poles through them, button the coats. The poles may be kept apart by strips of wood lashed to the poles at both ends of the bed formed by the coats.

**2** Make holes in the bottom corners of one or more sacks and pass strong poles through them keeping them apart as in the first improvising.

**3** Tie broad bandages at intervals to two strong poles.

**4** Spread out a rug, piece of sacking, tarpaulin or a strong blanket, and roll up two strong poles in the sides.

Otherwise, a hurdle, broad piece of wood, door, or shutter may be used. Rugs, clothing, hay or straw should be placed on it and covered with a piece of stout cloth or sacking which is useful for taking the casualty off the stretcher.

Always test an improvised stretcher before use.

## RULES FOR CARRYING CASUALTIES ON STRETCHERS

As a general rule, the casualty is carried feet first. The exceptions are:

**1** When going upstairs or uphill with a casualty whose lower limbs are uninjured.

**2** When going downstairs or downhill with a casualty whose lower limbs are injured.

**3** When carrying a casualty to the side or foot of a bed.

**4** When loading an ambulance.

### To cross uneven ground

If possible, the stretcher should be carried by four bearers and kept as nearly level as possible. This can be done, and the casualty prevented from falling off, by each bearer independently adjusting the height of the stretcher as necessary. Over very uneven ground for a short distance, the four bearers should face inwards.

### To cross a ditch

The stretcher is lowered near the edge of the ditch. The two front bearers get into the ditch and all four bearers lift the stretcher together, moving it forward until the rear handles rest on the edge of the ditch. The rear bearers get into the ditch and the stretcher is then moved forward on to the ground and rests there while the rear bearers get out of the ditch.

**To cross a wall**

Avoid crossing a wall, if possible, even if it means a longer distance. If there is no gap, the stretcher is lifted on to the wall so that the front runners are just over it, and the stretcher held level by the ear bearers while the front bearers cross the wall. All bearers then lift together and the stretcher is moved forward until the rear runners are clear of the wall, the stretcher being held level by the bearers in front. The remaining bearers then cross the wall and the stretcher is lowered carefully from the wall. The stretcher is then carried in the usual way.

**To load an ambulance**

The loaded stretcher is lowered with the head one pace from the doors of the ambulance. The casualty will be loaded head first.

The bearers now stand to the stretcher. Nos. 3 and 4 at the head, and Nos. 1 and 2 at the foot.

On the command: Load, the bearers turn inwards, stoop, grasp the poles of the stretcher, hands wide apart, palms uppermost. They rise slowly, lifting the stretcher, holding it level at the full extent of the arms. Then they take a side pace to the ambulance, raising the stretcher evenly to the level of the compartment to be loaded. The front bearers place the runners in the grooves and then assist the rear bearers to slide the stretcher into its place and secure it. (If the slings have been used they should be kept with their stretcher.)

Many ambulances are provided with upper and lower berths. In such cases, the sequence of loading is: upper right, upper left, lower right, lower left.

If the ambulance to be loaded is of the single door type, it should be loaded in the following manner. On the command: Load, No. 4 will take up position inside the ambulance facing the stretcher and No. 2 will take up position opposite No. 3, with No. 1 between the handles facing the ambulance. Nos. 2 and 3 turn inwards and all three bearers lift the stretcher to the required height, move forward, and hand the head of the stretcher to No. 4, Nos. 2 and 3 moving backwards to assist No. 1 who will load the appropriate berth with No. 4.

**To unload an ambulance**

Two bearers take hold of the handles at the rear and gently withdraw the stretcher. As it is withdrawn, the other two bearers will take hold of the handles at the front and, taking the weight, lower it to the full extent of their arms. Then by side paces they march clear of the ambulance and lower the stretcher to the ground.

To unload an ambulance with a single door, Nos. 4 and 1 will enter the ambulance, with Nos. 2 and 3 on either side of the door to assist No. 1 to descend. The stretcher is then withdrawn from the ambulance, and Nos. 2 and 3 receive the head of the stretcher from No. 4. Then the stretcher is carried clear of the ambulance and lowered.

# CHAPTER 14

# Major Accidents: Hospital and Community Planning; Hazards of Nuclear and Allied Radiations

The need for emergency planning by health service staff has long been recognised and the majority of hospitals have a disaster or major accident plan, which they would put into action should the need arise.

It is the responsibility of all nurses to know that plan and their part in it. They should know what to do whether they are off or on duty when the accident occurs. They must also know what is expected of them if there is an internal catastrophe, that is flooding, burning or bombing of the hospital itself. They must know how to mobilise help, evacuate patients and prevent the disaster from spreading. Each hospital will have its own procedures in the event of such happenings and also have contacts within the community to increase their efficiency and to confine the disaster. It is important that all hospital emergency plans are coordinated with those of other hospitals and appropriate statutory services and voluntary agencies in the area. Again, nurses should acquaint themselves with these plans which will reflect the position of their hospital in relation to the overall community plan.

Whilst it is not the responsibility of nurses in training to assist in the development of such plans, an understanding of their underlying principles and of the factors which must take priority in any implementation, will help them to play a more useful and intelligent part when called upon to do so.

## Classification of major disasters

### Natural

**1** Climatic: cyclones, hurricanes, floods, drought.
**2** Seismic: earthquakes, volcanic eruptions.

**Manmade**

**1** Accidental

- **a** Transport—road, rail, water, airways.
- **b** Industry—machinery, chemicals.
- **c** Explosions—mines, gas, munitions.
- **d** Fires.
- **e** Biological—bacterial, viral, toxaemic.
- **f** Chemical—corrosives, toxic vapours, liquids.
- **g** Nuclear—radiation, contamination.
- **h** Sport.

**2** Premeditated

- **a** Terrorism.
- **b** Riots and civil disturbances.
- **c** War.

The United Kingdom rarely suffers from natural disasters, and major accidents in this country during the past 20 years or so, mainly have been those involving transport, for example, the Moorgate underground train, which overran the end of the line in a tunnel, or explosions either from bombs, such as the Old Bailey bomb explosion, or from chemicals or nuclear power, for example, Flixborough, where the explosion involved casualties over a 102 $km^2$. This section therefore concentrates on manmade major accidents, accidental and premeditated.

## PRINCIPLES OF PLANNING

It has been noted that most of the major accidents in this country produce between 15 and 20 casualties. Whilst many of our accident and emergency departments are capable of dealing with such numbers throughout the day, many will be overwhelmed if they all arrive at the same time and all require immediate treatment.

Because of the many variables, no one blue print can be produced for every hospital in the country, but certain principles have been established which will apply to all.

Plans must:

be recorded in a readily understandable way, published and made available to all those members of staff and others who are likely to be involved in putting the plans into effect be devised only after consideration of all influences which may demand modification. Therefore, they must be flexible to allow for the extent of the emergency as well as the availability of key personnel, supplies and facilities

be designed to balance the probable need or demand and the resources available or which can be mobilised

take into account two-way support and assistance involving other hospitals, organisations and the like

provide for the assignment of authority and responsibility within an organisational framework.

## PLANNING WITH OTHER SERVICES AND HOSPITALS

At the site of any major accident in this country, there will arrive members of the three emergency services—police, fire and ambulance.

The fire service deals with hazards such as fires and floods and it has the resources and trained personnel to rescue trapped victims.

The ambulance service is responsible for the initial treatment (first aid) and transport of casualties to hospital.

The police service controls the disaster site.

Each service will have its own control vehicle at the site to establish a link with its headquarters.

Hospitals are not always requested to provide staff to the scene of the accident, but often a member will be sent to obtain accurate and adequate information. Sometimes it is necessary for hospital personnel to treat patients at the site. Planning, therefore, should allow for both these functions and the necessary integration with other emergency services. Such coordination should be organised at regional, area and district levels of the National Health Service. Most emergency hospital services, in fact, will be based on the accident and emergency departments of District General Hospitals. Other hospitals may become involved where there are large numbers of casualties or where there are unusual problems such as radiation, toxic, chemical or infective hazards.

To begin with, conditions at the site of the accident are likely to be chaotic. Restoration of order depends largely upon communication—the right information getting to the right people quickly.

First, a command centre should be set up to make decisions and it is the job of reconnaisance to provide it with essential and accurate information upon which to base those decisions. At every stage—from accident site to the patients' final destinations—triage, a process of sorting (by grading or classification), is necessary. This will include grouping those who are too ill to be moved from the accident site to a hospital, without some life-saving procedure first being performed.

## COMPOSITION OF MEDICAL TEAMS

To provide information for the command centre is the main duty of the reconnaisance officer.The mobile team's duty is to provide triage (sorting) and resuscitation. The latter will involve care of the patient's airway, ventilation and circulation as well as the arrest or control of haemorrhage. If necessary, the giving of analgesia, sedation and the splinting of limbs may also be included. Such teams should, therefore, be composed of experienced anaesthetists, surgeons and nurses, the latter preferably with operating theatre expertise.

In the first place, one team only is likely to be sent out. If more are required, they should be drawn from other peripheral hospitals; the receiving hospital should not be further depleted of personnel.

### Team clothing

Team members must themselves be provided with protection from danger and exposure. Prominent retro-reflective markings on their persons are necessary, not only for their own safety but also so that they can be located when visibility is poor. Identification should be clear and large. Clothing should be strong, weatherproof and all outside coverings should have many pockets. European green clothing is being used increasingly.

### Team equipment

Medical equipment should be familiar to the team members and similar to that which is currently in use at their own hospital. It should also be compatible with ambulance fittings and equipment. Each staff member should have a stout pair of scissors or a sheathed diving knife or both. All other equipment must be supplied in simple and easily managed packs or cases. Surgical instruments should be kept to the minimum range necessary for amputating a limb. Ketamine is the anaesthetic most frequently used under these conditions and should be made available to the teams. Ambulances will, in most instances, carry Entonox, suction apparatus, airway equipment, intravenous fluids and splints. The fire service will provide rescue equipment.

All packs, instruments and equipment belonging to each of the services should be robust, light and clearly labelled as to origin and content. Careful coordination, cooperation and collaboration at the planning stage will avoid duplications and omissions.

## CASUALTY CLEARING STATION

A casualty clearing station should be created near the control centre. Both will be as close to the scene of the accident as is consistent with safety. Sheltered protection from the elements and good lighting are essential features. The site must be made known to all rescuers, who should filter all casualties through it.

The main function of such a station is triage. Treatment carried out should be the minimum required to make the casualties fit for transportation to hospital. Anaesthesia and surgery are usually only required when victims have to be extricated from wreckage rapidly, either because of fumes, fire or flood. In these instances, a limb may have to be sacrificed in order to save a life. It is important to bear the crush syndrome in mind when dealing with patients who have been trapped under vehicles or rubble (see page 73).

Patient labels are essential and could conveniently follow the pattern of the specimen (Fig. 96). Coloured strips must be bright and large enough to be seen at a distance and preferably fluorescent. The label is attached to the patient with string, tied to a toe or finger. Sign boards with a corresponding colour code are erected on the disaster site and at the hospital so that patients may be brought to the sign boards (for collection by ambulance or for treatment) which match the colour of their labels.

Early location, certification and covering of dead people will contribute to the efficiency and efficacy of the rescue and resuscitation personnel.

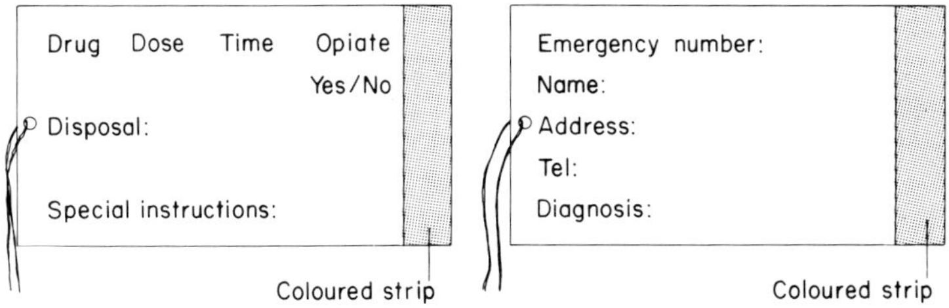


**Fig. 96** A patient label. The strip is colour-coded to various conditions: red—urgent resuscitation to save life (major injury); yellow—requiring hospital or medical attention but not so urgently (less serious injury); green—'walking wounded' requiring outpatient treatment (minor injury); black—dead.

Because communication between the accident site, the mobile unit, the casualty clearing station and the hospital can be a source of confusion and delay, appropriate VHF and UHF walkie-talkie radio sets and field telephones, together with experienced operators should be provided by the ambulance service.

## INITIAL RESPONSE OF THE HOSPITAL

Initial response of the receiving hospital should be in the form of augmentation of the accident and emergency department to deal with the precipitated arrival of a large number of casualties. Key roles will be taken by staff members available at the time. Duties attached to each role are usually summarised on an action card. This is either carried by the staff member at all times or is held at the command centre for collection when the need arises.

### The alert

The initial alert will be given by the local ambulance control station, who will have been warned by either their own staff, by the police or fire service or by a member of the public who has dialled the '999' emergency telephone call system. If, however, larger numbers of casualties appear in the department without warning, it is essential that the senior member of staff on duty at the time raises the alarm by him or herself immediately.

### Reconnaisance

Stress has been placed upon the value of reconnaisance in supplying information. This should include:

- estimates of the number of casualties
- types of injuries
- likely time of arrival at the hospital
- need for mobile medical teams
- any special information, that is, relating to toxic chemicals, radiation and the like.

This information should be sent to the hospital by the radio network of the ambulance service.

## PREPARATION AT THE HOSPITAL

A quick audit of the hospital bed-state will be necessary to establish the number of beds which are available. Some patients who are convalescent or waiting for investigations may have to be discharged quickly so that casualties can be admitted to their beds. Empty beds should be concentrated in one area in order to make the maximum use of resources—staff, equipment and facilities.

The accident and emergency department (including a reception area) and the operating theatres and other services such as radiology and blood transfusion, must also be alerted and made ready. Arrangements should be supervised by the senior member of the hospital staff who will receive from the command centre decisions relating to all necessary preparations. Another senior member of staff will be designated to supervise the streaming and sorting of patients as they arrive at the hospital. At this point, a simple classification is likely to be:

Group I Those needing urgent attention to safe life.
Group II Those requiring medical attention not so urgently.
Group III The 'walking wounded'.

It has to be remembered that because the less severely injured are usually the first to arrive, skilled staff and space must be reserved for Groups I and II at the outset of reception. Another member of staff—probably an anaesthetist—will supervise the carrying out of life-saving procedures and the preparation of those patients who require surgery.

### Control centre

A control centre should be set up near the accident and emergency department. Its responsibility will be to mobilise (and rotate as necessary for off-duty periods) appropriate medical, nursing and ancillary staff as well as personnel for the radiological and blood transfusion services.

Two other rooms will be needed; one for the care and counselling of relatives and friends of injured and dead people and another for the reception, selection, briefing and organisation of volunteers. Inevitably both groups will arrive in considerable numbers. The press and personnel of other media must also be catered for.

Volunteers who have received some training from one of the Voluntary Aid Societies (St. John Ambulance, St. Andrews and the British Red Cross Society) can be deployed very effectively, either by helping with routine work on the wards, or by listening, comforting and escorting the bereaved and anxious relatives of the victims. Members of the WRVS can also be invaluable in the latter role and will often be ready to supply hot drinks for helpers and the patients' families and friends.

## HOSPITAL MANAGEMENT

### Reception area

The area in which patients are received will be used for their classification, labelling and distribution to appropriate treatment zones. Documentation is also important at this stage. Some medical recordings will have been commenced at the accident site. Essential information will be that relating to drugs and fluids given and to trap or crush injuries. In the reception area these notes must be incorporated in the hospital records. All subsequent observations, treatment and the patient's hospital destination should also be entered in simple, concise language. A duplication system is necessary in order to provide the police information system with the data they require.

Patients with injuries which can wait should be transferred to another area. Volunteers can often be useful in providing the 'listening ear' so many of the victims will need.

## Resuscitation area

The resuscitation area should be a well-lit and open space. Its function is to provide life-saving practices and to prepare for surgery those casualities who require operations. It should also facilitate the admission to wards of those patients whose conditions have become stable. Theatre lists will probably be prepared by the senior anaesthetist supervising this area, but he may require specialist advice in the management of burns and certain other injuries such as those to the face, neck, chest, eyes and those affecting the vascular system. The main tasks of nurses working in this area is to carry out those life-saving procedures within their area of competence and to provide reassurance to their patients. In doing so, they will contribute to the creation of an atmosphere of confident and competent calm.

## Operating theatres

One of the aims of triage is to avoid the blocking of theatres with patients who require surgery for minor injuries, and who may arrive first, in the reception area. A separate theatre is often set aside for them to be dealt with after the patients with major problems have been treated.

## Wards and intensive care units

Wards and intensive care units should be organised to follow up the initial care given to patients in the accident and emergency department as well as those sent down from the operating theatres. It is important to re-check that the patients' destinations have been recorded, as it is very easy to 'lose' patients under these conditions. If this datum has been omitted, the information service should be notified. All requests for information from the communications media should also be referred to this service. No information should be given to any member of the media by the nursing staff.

## Radiology department

Radiological assessment is often required for the correct management of casualties. Bottlenecks of traffic must be avoided and it is another function of the triage officers to establish, and adhere to, strict criteria for priority X-rays. They may also report on the radiographs. In operating theatres especially, the use of image intensifiers defer the need for developed films.

### Blood transfusion department

Included in the hospital's major accident plans should be policy regarding the cross-matching of blood. A designated member of staff should supervise the flows of blood samples collected from the injured and the delivery of the requested blood and blood products. Most initial replacements of blood volume can be carried out using plasma substitutes. If they are used, the fact must be recorded on any request sheets as it is important that the laboratory staff know.

## EFFECTS OF MAJOR ACCIDENTS ON HEALTH SERVICE PERSONNEL

Major accidents can produce situations in which staff have to work long hours under great pressure and in distressful circumstances. A period which is acceptable for efficient and safe functioning should be identified, made known and adhered to. If amendments to the roster are necessary, these should be recognised and dealt with quickly by the appropriate senior member of staff.

Some disasters involve the hospital services in exceptional workloads for days or even weeks. Delayed primary suturing of wounds, orthopaedic work and staged plastic or reconstructive surgery can provide implications for the elective work of hospitals and may affect staffing schedules. Cooperation, understanding and flexibility is called for from each member of staff. Sometimes, the rehabilitation of both hospital and community can be protracted and arduous. Encouragement will be needed by everyone and an *esprit de corps* will be essential to the good morale of all services.

## TESTING OF EMERGENCY PLANS

With today's rapid turnover of hospital staff, it is vital that their knowledge of the hospital's disaster plan is tested at certain intervals. Each individual member of staff should be able to demonstrate knowledge of his or her specific role. Random tests may be made and some parts of the plan, such as the initial preparation of the accident and emergency department, can be tested in isolation.

In this way evaluations can be carried out of the staff training programmes and also of the logistical plans. Identified deficiencies and difficulties should be dealt with at once, amendments made and the plan re-tested as soon as possible. Only by doing so, can the confidence and competence of each staff member be ensured.

## FIRE OR OTHER DISASTER AT THE HOSPITAL OR HEALTH INSTITUTION

Most fires are a result of carelessness. It is the responsibility of hospital administrators and health workers to do all within their power to prevent fire and other disasters from occurring in their place of work.

If one does occur, early detection, prevention of spread, prompt extinguishing and, when necessary, quick competent evacuation of patients and staff are all vital activities. Fire regulations vary from hospital to hospital but must be known by all.

Fire protection requires planning, instruction in the use of fire-fighting equipment, frequent fire drills and inspections and strict adherence to laid down regulations. The entire staff of any health institution should be familiar with measures of fire prevention and control. One individual should have overall responsibility for that programme.

Each member of the hospital personnel—including students and learners—should know the following procedures in case of fire:

- how to raise the alarm
- how to use fire extinguishers
- how to remove patients to a place of safety
- how to protect the nose and throat from smoke

It is impossible to say what one should do first when a fire has been discovered; it depends entirely upon the circumstances. In most instances, sounding the alarm would be appropriate but if one patient or bed is on fire, or both are, it would be more sensible to first extinguish it with a blanket or with water from the nearest source. If oxygen is being used, that must be turned off at once. If the fire is noticed in an empty room, some distance away from a telephone or fire alarm, the first thing would be to close the door of that room to confine the flames.

If trapped in a burning building, it should be remembered that most fire deaths occur from the inhalation of smoke and toxic vapours. Certain procedures should be followed therefore to prevent flames and smoke from reaching unaffected areas. These include:

closing all doors and vents

plugging all cracks with wet cloths

opening windows from time to time for ventilation, but not if smoke and hot air are drawn into the room by doing so

Procedures to be followed for removing a bed-fast patient should be devised, known and rehearsed. The one most usually followed is to pick him up on the underblanket or mackintosh under the mattress and drag him along the floor and to a place of safety (Fig. 97). Firemen have belts which they can strap under a mattress and remove the patients in a similar way.

In order to prevent panic, it is vital for the nursing staff to maintain coolness and calm. The senior nurse on duty must quickly instruct others in their priorities and responsibilities whilst simultaneously raising the alarm for help.

Treatments for asphyxia and burns are given on pages 79 and 187.

## HEALTH HAZARDS OF NUCLEAR AND ALLIED RADIATIONS

By mid-1980 local authorities in Great Britain were urged by Her Majesty's Government to overhaul their civil defence plans particularly in relation to nuclear and allied radiations. These local plans should be known to all doctors and nurses working in the area.

### Sources

The natural radiation to which mankind has been exposed comes from certain radioactive elements which have always existed in the earth and atmosphere, although their presence has been recognised only for a few decades. These, and cosmic radiation, are usually referred to as 'background radiation'.

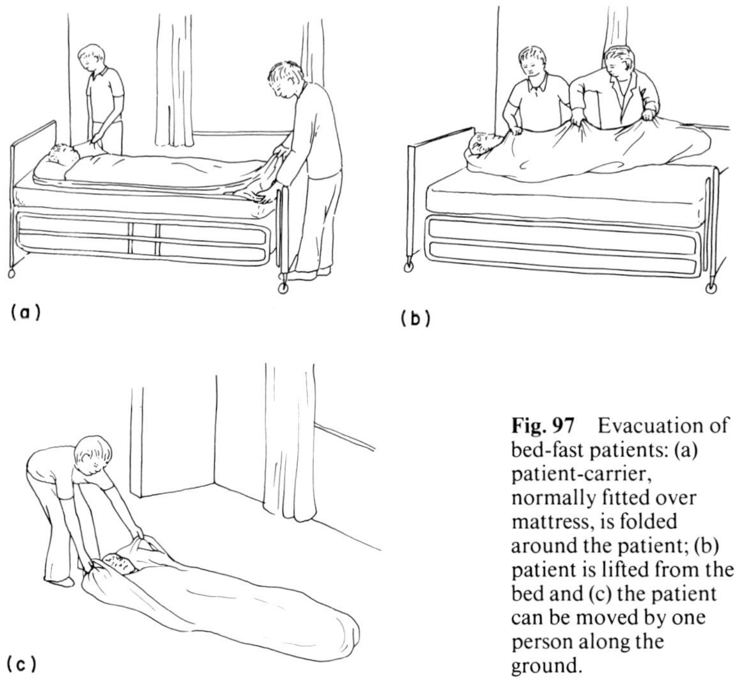


**Fig. 97** Evacuation of bed-fast patients: (a) patient-carrier, normally fitted over mattress, is folded around the patient; (b) patient is lifted from the bed and (c) the patient can be moved by one person along the ground.

Man himself has added to these sources and the extra radiations are derived from:

**1** The use of various forms of radiation in medicine and industry, for example, X-radiography and luminising.

**2** The isotopes and elements produced in nuclear reactors and by the explosion of nuclear weapons.

## Types

Radioactivity is the word used to describe the spontaneous disintegration of certain atoms into other forms, with the emission of radiations. Basically there are four types:

**1** Alpha radiation, consisting of particles of high energy, but with a power of penetration of less than one-tenth of a millimetre in human tissues. Because of their poor powers of penetration these particles are not considered a serious external health hazard but, if ingested, they become a serious danger to health. An alpha particle is positively charged, and is similar to the nucleus of the helium atom, that is two protons, two neutrons.

**2** Beta radiation, consisting of electrons (the orbital particles in the atomic structure) which carry a negative charge of electricity. Powers of penetration are poor, and the range of about a metre in the air. Again, the main health hazard is internal. If, however, the skin is bombarded for a sufficiently long period, burns will result.

**3** Gamma rays and X-rays, electromagnetic radiations of ranging energy, with high powers of penetration and capable of irradiating the whole human body uniformly.

**4** Neutrons, consisting of uncharged particles (a component of the nucleus in the atomic structure), with very high powers of penetration; able to irradiate the whole body. A characteristic of neutrons released during a nuclear explosion is that they are capable of inducing radioactivity and can, of course, present immense problems in decontamination after the detonation.

### 'External' and 'internal' radiation

Radiation from natural or artificial sources may be regarded as 'external' or 'internal' according to whether the source is outside or inside the body. External radiation refers to those radiations that strike the body from such sources as radioactive fall-out from a nuclear explosion or the radiation released at the time of detonation of a nuclear weapon. At the other end of the scale this also includes cosmic radiation.

'Internal' radiation arises from the ingestion or inhalation of radioactive materials into the body, an example being strontium 90 incorporated into the bones after ingestion or inhalation.

## Effects on living tissues

Millions of cells in the tissues of the human body die and are replaced every day. The effect upon cells exposed to radiations varies considerably (Table 5):

**1** With massive, whole-body doses of radiation there is gross tissue

**Table 5** The effects of differing amounts of whole-body penetrating radiation

| Dose (in up to 1 week) rads | Effect |
|---|---|
| Up to 150 | No acute effects. Serious long-term hazard, e.g. shortening of life-span: changes affecting the mutation rates. |
| 150–250 | Nausea and vomiting within 24 hours. Minimal incapacity after two days. |
| 250–350 | Nausea and vomiting in under four hours. Symptom-free period for 48 hours. Some deaths will occur in two to four weeks. |
| 350–600 | Nausea and vomiting in under two hours. Many deaths in two to four weeks. Incapacity prolonged. |
| 600+ | Nausea and vomiting almost immediately. Death within about a week. |

*Source:* Skeet M. (1977) *Manual for Disaster Relief Work.* Edinburgh: Churchill Livingstone.

destruction and the damage done is too great to enable effective repairs to be carried out. If this occurs, death is almost certain.

**2** With smaller doses of whole-body radiation the effect would be probable recovery of the individual but with certain malfunctions occurring either later in life or, perhaps, even in later generations caused by surviving irradiated cells eventually dividing, for example cancerous growths in later years and increases in the mutation rate.

Recovery from radiation exposure does occur but it must be understood that doses received are cumulative. However, the eventual outcome will depend upon:

**1** The amounts received and the rate at which they are received.

**2** The time between doses.

**3** The type of radiation and the area or part of the body exposed.

For example, an exposure of 5 rads per year for workers handling radioactive substances is permitted. The total amount which they are allowed to receive during a working life of 40 years is 200 rads. This is the maximum and, although a dose of 200 rads is received, the time taken to receive it is so long that no ill effects would be felt. If, however, the worker was to receive, two exposures of 100 rads within a relatively

**Table 6** Natural history of exposure of human beings to 400 rads as an immediate dose of whole-body penetrating radiation

| History | Symptoms | Duration |
|---|---|---|
| Exposure | None | |
| Interval | None | Lasting three hours |
| Initial symptoms | Nausea and vomiting | Lasting 12 to 24 hours |
| Interval | Period of indefinite symptoms | Lasting about a week |
| Radiation sickness | Loss of hair, loss of appetite, fever, inflammation of throat, haemorrhage, death of about 30 per cent commencing two weeks after exposure, those recovering will have prolonged incapacity | Beginning about 10 days after exposure |

*Source:* Skeet M. (1977) *Manual for Disaster Relief Work.* Edinburgh: Churchill Livingstone.

short time, clinical effects might become apparent. Some ill effects would almost definitely be felt by the individual at the time of the exposure. Symptoms would then appear either days or weeks later, similar to those shown in Table 6. Although radiations cannot be detected by any human sense, it is possible that exposure to large doses of highly penetrating radiation may be felt by the individual at the time of exposure. On the other hand, exposure over a longer period may or may not be felt.

## Management of victims

The management of radiation victims is dependent upon local conditions. Nevertheless it should be possible to plan the organisation

**Table 7** First aid and further treatment in radiation accidents

| Type of accident | Dose (rem) | Symptoms/signs | First aid | Further treatment |
|---|---|---|---|---|
| Total or subtotal overexposure | 20–100 | None | Blood analysis | Sedation if necessary<br>1st week—daily blood and urine analysis<br>2nd week—biweekly blood and urine analysis<br>Admission to hospital |
| Total or subtotal overexposure | 100–1000 | Nausea, vomiting, blood disorders within 4–6 hours, marrow syndrome | Blood analysis every 2 hours, sedation | |
| Total or subtotal overexposure | > 1000 | Shock, diarrhoea, gastrointestinal syndrome, cardiovascular and CNS syndrome | Blood analysis, treatment of shock, sedation | Admission to hospital, symptomatic treatment |

| Type of accident | Dose (rem) | Symptoms/signs | First aid | Further treatment |
|---|---|---|---|---|
| Regional overexposure | – | Redness, swelling | Blood analysis, sedation, treatment of pain | Possible admission |
| Regional contamination and injury | – | Wound | Irrigation of wound, promotion of bleeding | Treatment of wound |
| Regional contamination without injury | – | None | | |
| Inhalation/ ingestion/ percutaneous absorption | – | None | Gastric lavage, laxative | Possible admission |
| Combined effects | – | Dependent upon injury | Life-saving measures | Dependent upon nature of injury |

*Source:* Baillie T. W. & de Boer J. (1980) *Disasters: Medical Organisation.* Oxford: Pergamon Press.

so that selection for further medical care takes account of symptoms as well as exposure. In Table 7 an attempt has been made to relate the seriousness of the radiation accident with appropriate first aid and the later necessary medical treatment.

# CHAPTER 15

# Psychological Emergencies

Psychological emergencies can be defined as 'the results of things which suddenly upset or disturb one's normal life behavioural pattern, with temporary or long-lasting effect'.

Although, for ease of presentation they could be described in three groups—minor, moderate and major—the effects on people vary greatly in depth, with circumstances and with the strengths and weaknesses of individuals.

The causes of psychological emergencies are generally environmental, that is, those things which affect a person from without, and could arise from climatic, social and familial conditions, for example, a road accident with a car out of control due to icy conditions (climatic); a burglary at home (social–antisocial); the death of a near relative (familial). Seeing the road accident about to occur, hearing the crash, could be said to have a physical cause.

## STRESS

Stress which arises through the special senses—sight, hearing, touch, smell and taste—is physical and exogenous. If the cause of the emergency arises from within, for example, when severe pain is suddenly experienced, it could be described as physical and endogenous.

The effects of stress on individuals often result in unusual behaviour. A person's performance may be quite bizarre in character. For example, a man in need of help enables his own coping mechanisms to overcome the situation. Coping mechanisms to deal with awkward and stressful emergencies may be innate, but many more are learnt throughout life. Strategies are developed to avoid painful conditions, but as anxiety increases the usual coping system becomes ineffective and appears to leave the individual temporarily, abandoning him to his unprotected feelings.

The basic human needs of security, love, belongingness and fulfilment of potential are met emotionally and socially as an individual develops into maturity. Encounters with stress, however, interfere with the gratification of these needs and create psychological disequilibrium within an individual.

The helper who wishes to become effective in providing care for those in need might have to change her or his own behaviour. It is necessary to develop self-awareness and to examine sources of one's discomfort. As no one individual is an island it is important to know one's own self by asking questions:

How do I feel about this?
Where am I in all this?
What do I want from this?
Why do I feel . . . ?

Even so, the ability to assess, understand and empathise is not learnt easily, although some of it may be innate. A great amount has to be cultivated. One of the best ways of learning and adding to one's skills, is to listen and to watch. Not everyone expresses feelings in the same way, and every situation is different.

To assist, the helper must try to discover what has happened, from personal observation, from what others have told her or him, and from as much information as possible that can be gained about any upheaval or recent event. By moving in a competent and confident way all efforts to help will probably decrease the patient's anxiety and increase the acceptance of the need for care. If the patient can talk, state his or her name, describe the incident, provide information, the amount of the stress can be estimated by an observant first-aider. An experienced helper can also gain much from a person's non-verbal behaviour. The result of the emergency has to be recognised and the overdramatisation or intentional uncooperativeness on the part of the patient, noted. Reactions to crises are determined by past experiences and a lifetime of coping successfully and unsuccessfully with stress, but they cannot be predicted entirely for any one individual in a given emergency situation.

**Categories of assistance**

**1** Masterly inactivity—leaving the person alone.

**2** Activity—providing help to the person, seeking out friends or family or both, entertainment, being with the person for a meal, or even walking the dog.

**3** Verbal assistance—explanation, reassurance, advice.

**4** Non-verbal assistance—bodily contact, listening, body language (response without contact).

However well trained, however much experienced, the best helper will only be really successful after developing a non-judgemental attitude in her or his caring work. Such an attitude is essential to establishing a helpful relationship with a person who is experiencing the discomfort and pain of a psychological emergency.

## Minor stress

**Unstable psychological equilibrium**

For a child, prevented from attending school sports because he develops measles, the disappointment can be so great as to bring about tears and tantrums, when he or she is confined to home.

The cancellation of a plane for a party of adults resulting in an over-night delay is disturbing and the usually respectable quiet party becomes a restless, talkative, questioning group with loss of reserve and patience.

For these examples of minor stress, intervention to help is usually unnecessary. The fact that the child has an outburst and the travellers talk together is generally sufficient for all of them to draw on their coping strategies.

**Recognition**

Observing the increased alertness, the attentiveness of the individual, the free talking about the emergency, restlessness, repetitive questioning, and even perhaps telling a similar story or joking aid in recognising minor stress. It is often seen in bystanders at a road traffic accident, when people are eager to describe what they have seen and they question one another about it.

The assistance that is needed is the redirection of the bystanders. Giving them messages to send, or jobs to do, often is sufficent and effective.

## Moderate and severe stress

In order to describe moderate and severe stress and the ways of helping those who suffer, enlarging on the idea of a road accident is useful.

A motor coach, filled with holidaymakers, developed a mechanical fault, got out of control down a hill and crashed into a wall. The people involved were:

the driver, *Mr Mobile,* who was killed

the passengers, *Mr* and *Mrs Standing* who were injured, and several passengers who were 'shaken up'

the bystanders in the village

absent relatives and friends

*Mr Mobile,* the driver, had been pronounced dead. He was therefore beyond any help.

The others who are listed were suffering in different ways from psychological disequilibrium due to the serious accident. The uninvolved bystanders showed minor stress and their changed behaviours have already been described.

### Recognition of moderate stress

Among the passengers on the coach who were 'shaken up' were *Miss Lowring, Mr Highcatch* and *Mrs Middleton.*

*Miss Lowring* was discovered sitting quietly inside the coach and appeared to be unable to talk or respond in any way. When she was encouraged to move, she was found to have a pulse rate faster than normal, yet she was trembling. On going down the steps of the coach, she vomited, and then fainted.

*Mr Highcatch* was aggressive: he argued loudly with the policeman who was called to the scene and threatened to strike one of the passengers who tried to quieten him. He perspired freely and was breathing rapidly for several hours after the accident.

*Mrs Middleton* ran up and down the coach before she was persuaded to get off. She gave orders to the people left in the coach but there was no connection between any of her commands, and she failed to see whether they were understood, let alone carried out.

All three were unable to concentrate on anything that was asked of them. They were unable to follow directions, give a helping hand to others, or even lift up a few pieces of hand luggage.

Other passengers, who were not named, felt very sick when they reached home, and several had diarrhoea.

**Unstable psychological equilibrium due to moderate stress**

All the reactions mentioned can be brought about by unstable psychological equilibrium. At the same time those affected may have quite profound physiological effects. *Mr Highcatch* and *Mrs Middleton* demonstrate the 'fight or flight' theory of disturbed behaviour.

**Recognition of severe stress**

*Mr* and *Mrs Standing* were trapped under the seats. They later said that they thought of themselves as being in acute danger—their lives and their security and their future mobility were threatened. *Mr Standing* tried to tell his wife that they were 'in a bad way' and that it would 'take a long time to get right again', and he kept repeating this over and over again whilst in no way attempting to move himself.

*Mrs Standing* was apparently unable to hear her husband's words. She kept struggling to free herself, and she became more and more agitated as she discovered she was held firmly in between the seats. Whilst waiting to be freed she became disorientated and confused. Even her husband could not understand what she was saying.

Whilst all this was going on, none of the bystanders or the helpers had noticed that a young girl had slipped away from them. She too had been a passenger on the coach. She was brought back to the vicinity of the coach, screaming, crying, kicking out at people and appeared quite wild. She had fled in panic.

To assist *Miss Lowring, Mr Highcatch* and *Mrs Middleton,* it was essential that the helpers approached them in a calm, confident and competent manner. Attempts were made to get these three people to describe what had happened and to say how they felt. This helped a little in getting them to come to terms with the emergency. *Mrs Middleton* began to talk, and to cry, and her distress was alleviated in a short time. *Mr Highcatch* was more difficult to deal with. After about 15 minutes the policeman managed to persuade *Mr Highcatch* to write out his personal details and this simple task, by redirecting his thoughts, helped to re-establish his feelings of control and usefulness.

*Miss Lowring* required more active help. On recovering from the fainting attack it was necessary to talk quietly to her and the helper was able to describe how she thought she would feel in similar circumstances. Gradually *Miss Lowring* responded to the warmth of the helper's voice and became less withdrawn.

*Non-verbal communication*

One of the male helpers went to sit next to *Mr Standing* and by placing an arm around his shoulders he conveyed his concern and a willingness to help. Another helper held *Mrs Standing*'s hand and by just sitting on the floor next to her was able to bring about a measure of relief.

*Physiological changes*

Further complications and injury were avoided by making the *Standings* as comfortable as possible, although at first it looked almost impossible. The first-aider had to make it clear that he wanted to help and understand, and it was necessary to say this and to show it several times to get the message across. However skilled the helper might be, members of the *Standings'* family, or their friends, had they been available at the time, would probably have relieved the discomfort in less time.

When it was thought that *Mr Standing* had improved, his helper moved to assist *Mrs Standing. Mr Standing* then started to breathe rapidly, he became short of breath, said he felt very weak and dizzy, and that he was going to faint. His helper quickly returned to him, and managed to find a paper bag for him to breathe in and out of, in order to increase the amount of carbon dioxide in the air being breathed, and eventually his breathing returned to normal and the hyperventilation (overbreathing) stopped.

*Assistance in panic*

The girl had lost control of herself completely. The helpers had to intervene. She could not see the danger she was in and was unable to appreciate the efforts to help her. The people seemed to frighten her more. One helper had to restrain a person standing by from striking her, and another from dousing her with water. She was taken to a quieter environment and further care was given.

It was remembered that the words of the helpers are not always heard by a person in panic, but non-verbal messages, rate of speech, tone of voice, often were understood, so the helpers acted accordingly. Had the panic not been checked, it could have been communicated to some of the other people standing around and the girl herself could have become thoroughly exhausted. It is an extremely overpowering reaction to stress.

*Response to care*

As the individuals responded to the care given to them, their usual coping mechanisms came into play. Several of them then felt acutely embarrassed—even ashamed of themselves. They were told that most individuals have strong emotional reactions to emergencies and their actions were not uncommon, especially in people who narrowly escaped physical injury. They were asked to keep in touch with the members of their familes, or friends, and not to be alone for hours at a time, if it could be avoided.

*Reactions to death*

*Mr Mobile* was killed in the accident. When *Mrs Mobile* was told, she just could not believe it. She attempted to deny the seriousness of the accident, discount reports of it and could not come to terms with the loss of her husband. Later, she said that she felt sick 'in waves' with a choking feeling in her throat, an empty feeling in her stomach, and she had difficulty in breathing. At first she was angry with the person who told her, and then with the coach owners for not keeping the vehicle in perfect condition. She felt guilty and had mixed strong feelings as if she had failed her husband in some way and yet angry towards him too for having abandoned her. She felt like this for several weeks, not realising that they were the reactions of a normal person in the grieving process.

*Mrs Mobile* was in great need of help. Her immediate family gave her the psychological support she needed. They did not forcefully confront her with the reality of the loss, nor did they try to reinforce the rejection of the reality. They answered her questions honestly and empathetically.

As with a great number of people, *Mrs Mobile*'s bereavement period lasted a long time. It was nearly 2 years before she was able to accept the loss and reorganise her life. Her family and then her friends supported her in a variety of ways throughout this period.

*Threatening suicide*

Many factors contribute to self-destructive behaviour: generally those concerned suffering from depression related to recent bereavement, loss of self-esteem, prolonged physical illness; but also often disruptions in family life, economic distress, social isolation are part of the problems overwhelming individuals.

*Mr Mobile*'s driver-partner, a man in his fifties, just could not accept the situation. Business had been bad for a long time, and he had lost a lot of money. He had threatened to commit suicide more than once, when his wife left him for another man.

Fortunately his son had remembered all this. When he saw his father upset by the accident, giving away his possessions and avoiding people, he recognised these non-verbal clues and from his house across the road, he watched his father. The son knew about depression, hopelessness and helplessness—how the ordinary tasks become increasingly difficult to carry out, the increasing sense of fatigue—and the gradual social functioning changes, loss of appetite and loss of weight that unhappy people experience. He had the knowledge that when his father stated that he was 'going to kill' himself, he could not assume it was an idle threat.

*Mr Nightingale,* the son, was able to talk to his father. He moved in to live in his father's house for a time. He took away some of the obvious means of self-injury, and by showing him that someone cared he was able to convey messages of hope and help towards finding solutions to the main problem. By establishing such a good relationship he helped his father to cope and avoid death which was said, at first, to be the only way out of the problem.

*Psychotic behaviour*

None of the passengers in the coach showed psychotic behaviour. The roots of this inappropriate behaviour are in a variety of medical conditions or are induced by drugs. Prolonged psychological disequilibrium can precipitate a psychotic state in which patients misperceive or misinterpret the realities about them. They can become disruptive and be disturbing to others. They are obviously not meeting their basic safety needs and a psychiatric emergency arises.

The immediate first aid is to protect the patient from self-harm or harming others, and try to get psychiatric help. The family and friends can provide background information and this helps to indicate whether immediate medical assistance is needed.

Psychotic patients show fear, rage, excitement and apathy, as moods and behaviours change. They can suffer from delusions stating that people wish to harm them, that peculiar things are happening to them, and also from hallucinations, hearing voices. They appear as confused, disorientated yet vague people. They have moods that swing from a state of complete withdrawal and mutism to being aggressively hostile and destructive—from talking incessantly to laughing and being constantly on the move. For the unfortunate individuals who are known to suffer in this way, external or internal stresses severely threaten them and the exaggerated behaviours described are their ways of coping with the stresses which they feel have been overwhelmingly imposed upon them.

### Assistance

In circumstances of stress, the helper must be calm, with a reassuring firmness, saying: 'My name is . . .' or 'I am . . .'; 'You seem to need some help, may I . . .?' It is helpful to ask the patient his or her name and then to use it. If possible the problem should be defined in a single statement and if moving about dangerously some words about it not being safe to be around at that place, may help. A remark like 'You seem to be upset, what's happened—can I help you?' does show that the helper wants to understand. Talking with the patient, trying to allay fear and beginning to make a basis for speaking truthfully is helpful.

There should be no attempt on the part of the first-aider to agree or disagree with the patient in his or her delusions. If one were to agree, the threats felt might be reinforced; if one disagrees, then aggression might be increased, and anger evoked. If the patient forces the helper to give an opinion, the helper could reply to the effect that she or he understands the patient truly believes what he or she is describing.

A change of environment which is less stimulating assists an over-reactive patient, who should be told where he or she is going, in a simple way, without any deception.

Physical restraint should be used only as a last resort, and then applied only by well-trained personnel. More than one nurse might be needed to restrain the patient effectively. The patient may react violently in self-defence and attempt to 'fight for his or her life'.

Until the patient can make decisions for himself, it will be necessary to involve relatives or legal authorities or both who can assume responsibility for the treatment of the patient, if only on a temporary basis.

## Sudden attacks of aggression

Many factors contribute to outbursts of aggression and violence in human society, some of which are social and biological. Some people appear to have inborn tendencies towards expressing violence. Antisocial and criminal behaviour is often associated with extrovert personalities, yet to some extent controlled by social conditioning.

Patients who are mentally ill, mentally handicapped or physically ill are always liable to show fear, frustration, anger or despair, but to this group has to be added those who have contempt for authority, those who are intolerant of previously accepted social patterns and those who have little regard for the worth of another human.

Social violence in all its forms increased in the latter half of the 1970s and has become an almost accepted part of daily living as can be seen by reading a daily newspaper or watching any day's television programme.

Patients suffering from hypoglycaemia, postepileptic states and head injuries may be very agitated in an accident and emergency department of a hospital, and unintentionally injure those who attend them. Whereas the patients with head injuries are often quite oblivious of their actions unless told afterwards, the others mentioned often apologise as they respond to care and treatment.

### Staff

All staff working in an accident and emergency department must be prepared, protected and to some extent trained, as they face similar problems to their colleagues working in psychiatric hospitals. Sudden outbursts of aggression may come from patients, relations, friends or even intruders.

Nurses must always be on guard, aware of their limitations and aware of their actions. In the event of an outburst occurring outside the hospital where no help may be forthcoming, then it is preferable to leave the patient and seek further aid. As aggression and violence have to be dealt with quickly and positively, the nurse who first receives the patient has to be speedy in deciding whether to call the doctor immediately or whether the patient is able to wait, in turn along with others. Those who are associated with child abuse, drug abuse, wife-beating or granny-bashing will need different care from that received by the spectators from a football match who may want to continue the discrediting of the opposing team and supporters. Tact, sympathy and a non-judgemental attitude are needed for the battered wife. A social worker's help may be needed for the injured granny who is so totally dependent for shelter and company that she cannot complain about the cause of her condition.

**Prevention of violence**

Prevention of violence or an outburst of aggression is of prime importance in an accident and emergency department of a hospital. It can sometimes be achieved by the skilful deployment of experienced staff by the nurse in charge, who is aware of the capabilities of the staff and, at the same time, aware of the behaviour patterns of some of the patients and people who attend the department. The skills of the nurses cannot be overemphasised as they try to recognise and cope with the fears and frustrations of the patients which might lead to violent outbursts.

When feeling vulnerable, a patient may attack another person, generally a member of the staff, in an attempt to defend himself or herself. The way with which the patient is dealt, will depend upon the length of the attack. The patient will continue to be violent if he or she continues to feel threatened.

The total management of violence and of patients who demonstrate violent behaviour is beyond the remit of this chapter, but it is possible for nurses working in accident and emergency departments to give considerable assistance and care to those in need.

**Assistance**

To assist the verbally aggressive person, the nurse must attempt to overcome the barrier to communication that has developed, by speaking quietly and kindly, without causing antagonism. It may be necessary to explain why an examination cannot be carried out at once and that 'having to wait' is regrettable but necessary. If a patient has sufficient insight, then just listening to what is being said or a clear explanation may be all that the nurse has to do to alleviate the frustration.

If the patient is suffering from drink, drug abuse or is mentally sick, the nurse will need to apply firm but gentle restraint and the doctor may order sedation. More than one nurse may have to help deal with the patient.

In order to deal with a person actually exhibiting aggression, an experienced nurse who is alert and quick to anticipate further aggression may move closely to the patient, because the closer the nurse is to an aggressive patient, the harder it is for the patient to do harm. When the patient learns that the nurse is in control, there is a tendency to calm down and the aggression stops. It is advisable for the nurse not to wear a wrist watch, cuff links, brooches, necklaces or rings or other jewellery which might cause injury.

**Self-inflicted violence**

Most accident and emergency departments have their 'regulars'. Some inflict violence on themselves by slashing their wrists, by burning, by overdosing, by swallowing a glass thermometer, by hammering a nail into themselves, or by mainlining with drugs. Open wounds may have become infected.

It is on these occasions that nurses may find it difficult to maintain a calm attitude. To have to carry out a stomach washout on the same patient two or even three nights running requires empathy and patience. The casualty doctor may seek the assistance of a psychiatrist to treat patients in this group especially if one has been specifically appointed to work in the department.

By working together as a caring team, the staff of an accident and emergency department can reduce tension and alleviate stress and prevent some situations from getting out of hand. The Joint Board of Clinical Nursing Studies certificate courses in Great Britain provide opportunities for registered and enrolled nurses to further their skills and make full use of available experience.

## SUMMARY

The *Helper* must be a person of some worldly experience and sophistication, who has a stable personality and a deep measure of inner security. Compassion to a high degree and a sincere desire to help those in trouble are needed. Also, it is necessary for the helper to have control over her or his emotions so that to some extent the involvement in the unhappiness of people that is essential, is not too great a psychological strain. It is of little use trying to rescue a drowning man, by diving into the water, if the would-be rescuer cannot swim.

The *Assistance* is by:

simple, direct communications
desire to help and wish to understand
seeking information about the emergency
enabling the use of existent coping skills
obtaining family and friends to provide support
working as a team member in the accident and emergency department of a hospital

### Other incidents likely to cause psychological emergencies

There are many incidents other than those previously mentioned in this chapter that are likely to cause psychological emergencies. These are listed under two categories: moderate and major.

**Moderate**

Spontaneous abortion.
Loss of a pet, especially with the young and old.
Examination failure.
Failure to get a job.
Being stuck in a lift.
Breaking off an engagement.
Change of religion.
Son sent abroad by a firm or to be a missionary.
Seeing cruelty to animals.
Opening the door to a frightened neighbour.

**Major**

Difficulties associated with childbirth.
Knowing that one's new baby is not normal.
Due to an accident, a child being deprived of its mother.
Violence in the family.

Being arrested by the police.
Loss of property by burglary.
Damage to property by fire.
Loss of job—redundancy.
Sudden loss of sight, hearing, limb and the like.
Onset of a 'stroke'.
Breakdown of marriage.
Being told of having developed malignant disease.
Being attacked in the street.

It is repeated that for ease of presentation, stresses could be described in groups, but the effects on people vary greatly with each incident, and the strengths and weaknesses of individuals. If these lists cause discussion among the readers, then the chapter will partly have achieved its purpose.

APPENDIX 1

# Recommended first aid equipment

## EMERGENCY FIRST AID CUPBOARD IN THE HOME

Nurses are often asked to give advice on the contents of a first aid cupboard in the home. The following list is recommended by the Voluntary Aid Societies:

| Item | Quantity |
|---|---|
| Adhesive tape, roll 2·5 cm × 5 m | 1 |
| Aspirin soluble, tablets, 300 mg | 25 |
| Bandages triangular | 4 |
| Bandages: conforming and open-weave, various | |
| Bowl, small plastic | 1 |
| Cotton wool absorbent, 15 g packets | 3 |
| Cream antiseptic (e.g., Savlon) tube (or antiseptic wipe, foil packed, e.g., Steriprep) | 1 |
| Dressings, adhesive (plasters) assorted | 24 |
| Dressings, adhesive, strip 6·5 cm × 90 cm packet | 1 |
| Dressings, sterile, small | 2 |
| Dressings, sterile, medium | 2 |
| Dressings, sterile, large | 2 |
| Dressing forceps, plastic (or tweezers) | 1 pair |
| Gauze, 90 cm × 0·5 cm packets | 3 |
| Lotion calamine, bottle (180 ml) | 1 |
| Liquid antiseptic (e.g., Savlon or Dettol), diluted ready for use 1 in 1000, bottle (180 ml) | 1 |
| Paracetamol (alternative to aspirin) tablets 500 mg. See note on aspirin dosage | 25 |
| Pins, safety, assorted | 12 |
| Scissors, blunt-ended, disposable, pair | 1 |
| Thermometer, clinical, oral | 1 |
| Torch | 1 |

**Note: All** sterile dressings should be placed in sealed plastic bags to keep them sterile and dry.

**Care** should be taken in the *dosage of aspirin* if given to infants and young children. Repeated doses should not be given except on medical advice. Some adults may be sensitive to aspirin.

Normal dosage is 2 tablets for an adult, 1 tablet for a 5–12 year old and ½ tablet for a 1–5 year old.

The cupboard should be readily accessible to adults, but locked or impossible to open by children.

A bathroom is not a suitable room for the first aid cupboard, as the storage atmosphere should not be damp.

**All** bottles and containers should be clearly labelled and should have tightly fitting (preferably screw) caps.

**Dressings** should be in small packs so that unused material is unlikely to be left over inadequately wrapped.

An item used should be replaced at the earliest opportunity.

## ON DUTY AT A SPORTING EVENT

The equipment the first-aider has at a sporting event will vary according to the event being covered, and the availability of other professional help. Personal equipment should be appropriate to the skill and training of the individual concerned.

A well-equipped first aid room will include a couch with blankets, good lighting, hot and cold running water, and a telephone with a list of appropriate telephone numbers for emergencies. The following list of useful equipment is by no means exhaustive:

| | |
|---|---|
| Ice and re-usable ice packs | A rigid stretcher |
| Sterile wound dressings | A selection of oral airways and one Brookes airway |
| Steristrips | Simple analgesics, preferably with non-steroidal inflammatory properties, e.g. Ponstan Forte (Parke Davis) |
| Cotton wool | Simple antacids such as Aludrox |
| Adhesive felt | Anti-diarrhoea preparation, e.g. codeine phosphate |
| Compression bandaging (Lyofoam, crepe) | Glucose supplements, e.g. Accolade (Nicalos) and salt supplements including Slow Sodium tablets (Ciba) |
| Tubigrip | |
| Triangular bandages | |
| Antiseptic, preferably Iodofore | |
| Splints, including padded wooden boards, air splints, spinal board and cervical collar | |

APPENDIX 2

# National Poisons Information Centres (British Isles)

**London**

Poisons Unit, New Cross Hospital, Avonley Road, London SE14 5ER, England.
*Tel* 01 407 7600 *Director* Dr R. Goulding

**Edinburgh**

Scottish Poisons Information Bureau, The Royal Infirmary, Lauriston Place, Edinburgh EH3 9YW, Scotland.
*Tel* 031 229 2477 Ext 2233 *Director* Dr A. Proudfoot

**Cardiff**

Poisons Information Centre, The Cardiff Royal Infirmary, Cardiff, Wales.
*Tel* 0222 492 233 *Director* Dr G. M. Mitchell

**Belfast**

Poisons Information Centre, Royal Victoria Hospital, Grosvenor Road, Belfast BT12 6BA, Northern Ireland.
*Tel* 0232 40503 J *Director* Professor R. Shanks

**Dublin**

Poisons Information Centre, Jervis Street Hospital, Dublin 1, Eire.
*Tel* 0001 745588 *Director* Dr J. A. Woodcock

**Note:** These centres only take enquiries from health professionals and not from the general public.

APPENDIX 3

# Selected Mortality and Related Statistics

## RABIES

The enforced quarantine of animals, domestic and other, entering the United Kingdom provides a safe control of rabies. Although non-existent in the UK, from 1946 to 1977 there were 13 deaths from the disease, which became notifiable on 3rd August, 1976. The deaths recorded from 1946 were of victims who had been bitten by rabid animals prior to their arrival in Britain. The following list shows the countries of origin, the number of patients and the year:

| | | |
|---|---|---|
| Greece | 1 | 1946 |
| Pakistan | 1 | 1947 |
| Afghanistan | 1 | 1955 |
| India | 1 | 1956 |
| Pakistan | 1 | 1963 |
| Indonesia | 1 | 1964 |
| India | 1 | 1967 |
| | 1 | 1969 |
| | 1 | 1975 |
| Gambia | 1 | |
| Bangladesh | 1 | 1976 |
| Pakistan | 1 | 1977 |
| India | 1 | |

## BITES AND STINGS OF VENOMOUS ANIMALS AND INSECTS

From 1970 to 1978, there were 24 deaths from bites or stings of venomous animals or insects. In the same years, other accidents caused by animals which resulted in death numbered 227. Twenty-seven of the bite-sting-accidental deaths in one year (1978) were assigned to: heifers (4); dogs, not rabid (3); and horses (20)—with 2 to bees alone.

## EXPOSURE FROM REDUCED TEMPERATURE

The category referred to as Effects of Reduced Temperature includes: Frostbite, Immersion, or Trench, Foot, and Excessive Cold, or Freezing. The deaths which occur in this category are registered as: accidental, suicide, undetermined and homicide. From 1970 to 1978, there were 537 deaths from reduced temperature of which 55 per cent were male. In 1976, 203 patients were admitted to hospital in this category; 156 survived the effects of reduced temperature.

## DRUGS, MEDICAMENTS AND ALCOHOL

In 1978, there were 617 deaths recorded as accidental poisoning by drugs, medicaments and alcohol: 286 (46 per cent) males and 331 (54 per cent) females.

The heaviest concentration of deaths from analgesics and anti-pyretics in males occurred between the ages of 15 and 29. Whereas, other sedatives, hypnotics and barbiturates accounted for 247 female deaths, with the heaviest concentration occurring between the ages of 40 and 79.

Alcohol poisoning (14·5 per cent of the total) was marginally higher in males, with a 62 per cent concentration of deaths occurring between the ages of 40 and 64. The greatest incidence of female deaths from alcohol poisoning occurred between the ages of 45 and 59.

## SOURCES

Department of Health and Social Security and the Welsh Office, 1977 Memorandum on Rabies, London, HMSO

Mortality Statistics, Series DH1 No. 5, 1977

Statistics of Infectious Diseases, Series MB2 No. 5, 1978

Mortality Statistics: Cause, Series DH2 No. 5, 1978

Hospital Inpatient Enquiry, Series MB4 No. 7, 1976

# APPENDIX 4

# Health and Safety at Work Act and the Learner Nurse

The learner nurse should be aware of the Health and Safety at Work Act 1974 as she or he is an employee of the hospital. As an employee she or he has certain rights to expect and duties to perform. Under the Act it is the duty of the employer to ensure the health, safety and welfare at work of all employees. This is usually set out as a written statement of general policy, and the general policy should include brief extracts from the Health and Safety at Work Act, which show what are the duties of management and what are the duties of staff. A health policy would usually give the name of the head of the department, the safety officer and the occupational health officer.

The nurse may belong to the trade union of her choice and as such should know the Safety Representative who is appointed by the union; the nurse should know that all hazards or accidents should be reported and she should know to whom they should be reported. Emergency telephone numbers are often stated on a health and safety policy, together with information as to where first aid is available, and it usually gives the location of the Occupational Health Department and how to use it.

The Health and Safety Policy may also give notes on protective clothing, when it is to be worn and why. Many nurses fail to realise that their own uniform is a protective clothing and should be treated as such. Within a hospital there are chemical substances of many types some of which when handled in bulk may be toxic or there may be an organic hazard. Reference should be made to these in the Health and Safety Policy and there may be Notes of Guidance telling people what is their duty for their own protection when handling such substances. Sometimes there are Codes of Practice published by the Health and Safety Commission under the Department of Employment. A typical

Code of Practice which applies to the hospital situation may be that on Ionising Radiations. Nurses who are engaged in handling these materials should have read the Codes of Practice and to know how to handle these potentially dangerous materials.

The Health and Safety Policy within a hospital will often give local advice as to hazards which occur in the hospital and to which the employee must take care even though there is not an official Code of Practice to govern activities in that department. For example there may be a specific procedure in a hospital with regard to the deposition of blades, scalpels and hypodermic needles. In many hospitals there is a special practice regarding these sharp pieces of equipment and the procedure for dealing with them should be rigorously followed.

The Health and Safety at Work Act states, 'It is the duty of the employer while at work to take reasonable care for the Health and Safety of himself [or herself] and of other persons'. Two other major hazards beset the hospital nurse, that of back injury due to lifting, and infections. Under the Health and Safety at Work Act therefore as it is the duty of the employer to inform the employee about the hazards, it is also the duty of the employer to provide instruction as to safe procedures to prevent the injury or disease, but it is also the duty of the employee, to learn the safe methods and to use the proper equipment provided.

It must be noted that under the Health and Safety at Work Act, *Health* refers primarily to the prevention of injury or disease arising during and directly due to the work of the employee. It is not therefore, a duty of the employer to provide an Occupational Health Service under the Act, but a good employer concerned with total health of the employee will do so.

# References

*A.B.C. of First Aid* (1972) London: British Red Cross Society.

BAILLIE T. W. & DE BOER J. (1980) *Disasters: Medical Organisation.* Oxford: Pergamon Press.

BIRCH C. A ed. (1971) *Emergencies in Medical Practice.* Edinburgh: Churchill Livingstone.

BURDEN G. & SCHURR P. (1976) *Understanding Epilepsy.* London: Crosby Lockwood Staples.

*First Aid:* the authorised manual of St. John Ambulance and St. Andrew's Ambulance Association and the British Red Cross Society. London.

MUCKLE D. S. (1978) *Injuries in Sport.* Bristol: John Wright.

PARCEL G. (1977) *First Aid in Emergency Care.* St. Louis: C. V. Mosby.

PROCTOR H. & LONDON P. S. (1977) *Principles for First Aid for the Injured.,* London: Butterworth.

RUTHERFORD W. H. *et al.* (1975) Surgery of Violence. *British Medical Journal,* **1,** 382, 443, 502, 559, 614, 667, 728; **2,** 25; **3,** 287.

SKEET M. (1977) *Manual for Disaster Relief Work.* Edinburgh: Churchill Livingstone.

SKEET M. & STROUD J. (1975) *Home Nursing.* London: Stanley Paul.

WILLIAMS J. G. P. & SPERRYN P. N. (1976) *Sports Medicine,* 2nd edition. London: Edward Arnold.

# INDEX